The Desire and Passion for a Child

T0384739

In this book, Patricia Alkolombre explores the desire for a child from a contemporary psychoanalytic perspective, and covers the questions raised in the face of new resources offered by reproductive medicine.

This volume reviews traditional psychoanalytic conceptualisations from the perspective of gender theories and analyses theoretical hegemonies related to the desire and passion for a child. Alkolombre discusses how the 'passion to have a child' is a key aspect of motherhood, characterised by emotional intensity, persistence, and self-sacrificial aspects.

The book is divided into three sections: Part One deals with the desire and passion to have a child, while Part Two focuses on the impact of reproductive techniques, as well as the ever-changing role of parenthood in the modern day. Throughout these fascinating chapters, clinical vignettes of both individual and couple analyses span topics such as mourning, the use of reproductive technology, the anonymity of gamete donors, enigmatic infertility, surrogacy, and abortion from an interdisciplinary perspective. The historical and cultural contexts of infertility are reviewed from a psychoanalytic angle in Part Three with the view of transcending the former androcentric perspective that has deeply influenced the maternal ideal and expectations of men. Alkolombre also proposes a new analysis of the Oedipus myth.

This book is vital reading for psychoanalysts, mental health professionals, teachers and students interested in contemporary parenting, motherhood, and infertility, as well as the theoretical analysis of the desire for a child.

Patricia Alkolombre, PhD, is Overall Chair of the IPA Committee on Women and Psychoanalysis. She is Training and Supervising Analyst of the Argentine Psychoanalytic Association (APA), a Postgraduate Professor at the APA-UBA master's degree and at other institutions in Argentina and abroad. She has written on infertility, the female body, femininity, masculinity, parenthood, psychoanalysis, and gender. She is a co-author of *Changing Sexualities and Parental Function in the Twenty First Century* (Karnac, 2017) and *Psychoanalytic Explorations of What Women Want Today: Femininity, Desire, and Agency* (Routledge, 2022).

Psychoanalysis and Women Series
Series Editor: Paula Ellman (previously Frances Thomson-Salo)

The *Women and Psychoanalysis Book Series* grew from the work of the International Psychoanalytical Association Committee on Women and Psychoanalysis (COWAP). Publications further the conversations on women, sexuality, gender, men, and psychoanalysis, and intersections with diversity and cross-cultural experience. We value written exchanges between psychoanalysis and related disciplines of gender studies, anthropology, sociology, politics, philosophy, arts, and activism. We encourage contributions from all regions, allowing for global perspectives and different creativities on topics relating to women, gender, and sexuality. The series editorial board is comprised of Paula Ellman (Editor-in-Chief, North America), Carolina Bacchi (North America) Sara Boffito (Italy), Lesley Caldwell (UK), Amrita Narayana (India), and Paula Escribens Pareja (Peru).

Titles in the series:

Changing Notions of the Feminine: Confronting Psychoanalysts' Prejudices Edited by Margarita Cereijido

When a Child has been Abused: Towards psychoanalytic understanding and therapy By Frances Thomson-Salo and Laura Tognoli Pasquali

The Courage to Fight Violence Against Women: Psychoanalytic and Multidisciplinary Perspectives By Paula L. Ellman

Changing Sexualities and Parental Functions in the Twenty-First Century: Changing Sexualities, Changing Parental Functions By Candida Se Holovko

Psychoanalytic Explorations of What Women Want Today: Femininity, Desire and Agency By Margarita Cereijido, Paula L. Ellman and Nancy R. Goodman

The Desire and Passion for a Child: Psychoanalysis and Contemporary Reproductive Techniques By Patricia Alkolombre

For further information about this series, please visit https://www.routledge.com/Psychoanalysis-and-Women-Series/book-series/KARNACPWS

The Desire and Passion for a Child

Psychoanalysis and Contemporary Reproductive Techniques

Patricia Alkolombre

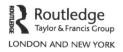
Routledge
Taylor & Francis Group

LONDON AND NEW YORK

Designed cover image: ssnjaytuturkhi / Getty Images

First published 2023
by Routledge
4 Park Square, Milton Park, Abingdon, Oxon OX14 4RN

and by Routledge
605 Third Avenue, New York, NY 10158

Routledge is an imprint of the Taylor & Francis Group, an informa business

© 2023 Patricia Alkolombre

The right of Patricia Alkolombre to be identified as author of this
work has been asserted in accordance with sections 77 and 78 of the
Copyright, Designs and Patents Act 1988.

British Library Cataloguing-in-Publication Data
A catalogue record for this book is available from the British Library

ISBN: 978-1-032-28406-4 (hbk)
ISBN: 978-1-032-27035-7 (pbk)
ISBN: 978-1-003-29671-3 (ebk)

DOI: 10.4324/9781003296713

Typeset in Times New Roman
by KnowledgeWorks Global Ltd.

Contents

Preface

The *Women and Psychoanalysis Book Series* developed from the work of the International Psychoanalytical Association Committee on Women and Psychoanalysis (COWAP). The IPA-Routledge series furthers global perspectives and different creativities on topics related to women, gender and sexuality, and psychoanalysis, considering intersections with diversity and cross-cultural experience.

In the present volume, Alkolombre presents an important contemporary discussion about motherhood and its vicissitudes, focusing on what happens when the desire to have a child becomes, as the author calls it, a passion. Alkolombre differentiates passion from desire while she proposes a more robust and complex understanding of the narcissistic axis present in the experience of motherhood and its particular attachment to sacrifice. The clinical vignettes move us from the theoretical to the practical, tracing the author's thinking about how these issues manifest in the analytic dyad.

Alkolombre reviews the different authors who have studied the theme of motherhood in the psychoanalytic field and beyond, inviting a broader understanding of how social expectations of motherhood have been transformed, even as the mandate that falls on women as mothers continues to prevail. By addressing the problematic of "passion," the author brings her readers to the centrality of the tension between the desire of the woman as a subject (with her own intrapsychic life, fantasies, and longings) and the social demand (installed also at an unconscious level). Perhaps one of the most central contributions that Alkolombre offers is the interwoven relationship between social and intrapsychic, and between clinic and theory when we work with mothers and mothers-to-be. The distinctions between the intrapsychic and the social, and between theory and practice are revealed as arbitrary constructions that she tries to unravel while differentiating the specificity of motherhood in opposition to fatherhood.

Alkolombre describes the impossibility of mourning for a child that one could not have, and links this mourning to the development of a passion for a child, which is imbued with passivity, contrary to what "passion" suggests. The clinical examples greatly enrich the understanding of this complex issue and invite us to reconsider culturally communicated prejudices and stereotypes. Current technological advances now allow women to actualise, while creating the perfect stage for women to display those inner conflicts. As she accompanies mothers traversing their journey of passion, Alkolombre hopes to transform passion into ordinary desire with a capacity for language and for fulfilling its aim. Alkolombre's *Desire for a Child. Passion for a Child: Reproductive Techniques in the Light of Psychoanalysis* is a brilliant and necessary book for all professionals working with women navigating the complex transition into motherhood.

The Women and Psychoanalysis Book Series Editorial Board represents all regions of the IPA with six editors collaborating as a team from Goa (India); London; Lima; Milan; San Francisco, CA; and Washington, DC. We are women writers and editors active in psychoanalysis both regionally and in the IPA. We encourage single author and multiple author book proposal submissions to our IPA-Routledge Book Series on topics of women, gender, femininity, and masculinity. We offer our close-up consultation and guidance in the crafting of the book proposals and throughout the writing and publishing process.

The Women and Psychoanalysis Book Series Editorial Board

Carolina Bacchi

Sara Boffito

Lesley Caldwell

Paula Ellman (Editor-in-Chief)

Paula Escribens Pareja

Amrita Narayanan

Introduction

The Desire and Passion for a Child brings psychoanalytic work into the field of reproductive techniques. It chronicles the questions provoked by different clinical presentations as a guide to provide thoughts and hypotheses on a topic linking bodies and desires through the longing for parenthood.

The *new order* of sexuality and procreation has modified the vicissitudes of the desire to have a child. We know that traditional ways of being born, that is to say, in the intimacy of a sexual relation, are over 2,000 years old, whereas those initiated by medical and technological intervention began in 1978.

New forms of cohabitation between genders also became legal, and power relations between men and women changed. Diverse filiation projects share a context of sexual diversity, including single parenthoods and homo-parentalities. These transformations upset symbolic references and affect the structures of symbolic systems governing the identification of subjects in relation to sexual and gender identity and procreation.

We are living in a unique historical period, a transition between generations born before and after the implementation of reproductive technologies. In the "pre-test-tube" era, men and women accepted natural fertility and adoption as the only means possible for having children. In contrast, current generations are immersed in changes brought about by the use of contraceptives and assisted reproduction. As witnesses of this historical transition, we have the privilege of exploring and explaining its repercussions on subjectivity.

To be born formerly meant to be born from the body of a woman who was that child's biological mother. Historically, women were always "in" their pregnancy. Today, the anchor point is not the woman's own body since a woman may now paradoxically be "watching" her pregnancy and her child's birth if she rents a womb. All these changes in parenting raise many questions in our clinical practice and our theories.

The place of the desire to have a child is the starting point of this book. This desire is linked to parental desires, the child's identity, and its origins.

DOI: 10.4324/9781003296713-1

Clinical work in this field is characterised by a significant absence: the child to come. It involves both disappointment and the promise of life.

The desire for a child has been addressed by different Freudian and post-Freudian perspectives and by gender theories. This topic raises questions concerning the vicissitudes of female and male infertility, living through the wait, the place of bodies, maternal and paternal roles, and women's plural desires with their clinical scenarios.

Technology enables us to explore the internal body and its secrets. Hence, the *predictable* body and the *transparent body* emerge through reproductive techniques which reveal their depth, their secrets, and the universe of meanings they acquire in each singular history.

The *passion for a child* is a certain type of maternity marked by emotional intensity and insistence on seeking pregnancy even at the cost of self-destruction. The distinction between desire for a child and passion for a child enables us to define clinical cases with self-sacrificial and thanatic aspects. Passion for a child is a desire that has become a need. It is the search for a child *at any cost*.

In our consulting rooms, we see patients who are undergoing assisted reproduction treatments. We analyse their conflicts, which involve the influence of what is foreign vis-à-vis the self in gamete donation, the issue of the anonymity of donors, and the psychic status of embryos, as well as the splitting of bodies in surrogate maternity, the problems underlying enigmatic infertility, and the effects of abortion on women's and men's lives. The psychic effects of these experiences observed in clinical work are described in clinical vignettes.

In this context, technology has introduced a *new order* in procreation, leading in turn to new filiation projects. At the beginning, the discovery of the contraceptive pill in the 1960s radically dissociated sexual activity from the arrival of children. Twenty years later, this equation was inverted by the implementation of assisted fertilisation techniques: it became possible to have children without having sexual relations.

At this point, we may ask ourselves whether the old can explain the new, and whether clinical work can be understood with the resources we have now or whether we are facing new representations in the reproductive field. What is certain is that maternity and paternity are no longer something well-known and familiar and have become a new alchemy in which bodies, fluids, and cells may be combined, substituted, and modified.

Therefore, it is very important for us to update and review these topics, which lead us to think and continue to question ourselves about what remains the same and what is changing in this field. The implementation of reproductive techniques has opened up new possibilities for access to parenthood, but has also led to new debates and questions about origins.

Cultural changes throughout history reveal androcentric and patriarchal perspectives on conceptions of maternity and paternity. Since the middle of the last century, the critical revision of sexuality, gender, and procreation has changed clinical practice and the way we may think about it.

These problems not only present theoretical-clinical challenges, but also touch on the analyst's theories and prejudices which may operate as obstacles. These experiences affect subjects' bodies and are intertwined not only in representations of the new and varied ways of being born today, but also in the extra-scientific field, such as children born as a result of techniques. In this regard, it is clinical work containing novel elements which exceed what was known until only 1978, confronting us with what is different in a field that unites bodies and desires in different kinds of parenting projects.

This book, like everything else, has a history, and in the course of its writing and rereading, it preserves, intact, the author's desire to transmit an experience, a personal perspective, and questions, to share them with others.

Part I

About the Desire and the Passion for a Child

Chapter I

Revisiting Desire for a Child

About women's desire

Desire for a child is a contemporary concept that has become a synonym for the *will to procreate* in everyday language. In our consulting rooms, we encounter novel experiences of men and women: new scenarios in the search for a child. Access to parenthood through reproductive techniques nowadays has broadened the possibilities. Furthermore, diversity is present in our clinical work in the shape of different family configurations: hetero, homo, and single parenthood. Diversity of desires is present in our practice.

Therefore, understanding of the subject matter of this book derives from a psychoanalytic theoretical frame that takes into account not only male-female binarism but also the perspective of diversity as in the *epistemology of complexity* (Morin, 1990). This epistemology accounts for the multidimensionality of our object of study. Complex thinking proposes a broad and comprehensive path beyond classic determinism. Thus, there is no pure chance or absolute determinism in itself, since this view admits the heterogeneous and the plural, thereby overcoming the dualism of binary thinking.

In this chapter, I propose that you delve first into the desire for a child in women. The desire for a child is the foundation on which the prehistory of unborn child will be constructed. It is also prehistory carved out of parental fantasy, their imago of the child's sexuality. From her childhood, every woman weaves complex patterns around motherhood, which are then inscribed in the act of procreation: to have a child by her father, her mother, her partner, or a self-procreated child. Motherhood is rooted in the female ego and in the most classic view of sexuality, which culminates in the arrival of a child. In his article on Femininity (1933) Freud further states that this desire is to give birth to a boy, influenced by the patriarchal ideology of that time and by the relation he had with his mother, Amalia Freud (Ferenczi, 1988).

In psychoanalysis, the desire for a child is the expression of unconscious motion. Every woman processes this desire in different ways. We may think about this desire through different approaches and reveal unconscious

DOI: 10.4324/9781003296713-3

desires hidden behind it. This desire emerges from childhood sexuality and is conceived within the intensity of the pre-oedipal and oedipal conflict. Since the pre-oedipal phase, the desire to have a child by her mother, to have a child with her mother, originates from mirroring: she wants to be a "mother" like her own mother.

The desire for a child is also rooted in oedipal conflict: to have a child by the father to compensate for penis envy. According to Freud, the girl's libido derives from the penis = child symbolic equation. In this new role, she renounces her desire for a penis by replacing it with the desire for a child. In this perspective, the desire for a child becomes the heir of the female castration complex, as well as a promise originated by the penis = child equation. We develop these issues in depth later.

I've often found myself thinking about women's path to develop their sexuality and how that path is walked with the promise and expectation of getting a woman's body. A body that during childhood is presented as "breastless and childless." For a girl, her mother's body is a reflection of a future self with "breasts and children." We discussed the anatomical difference between girls and women: an intra-gender difference related to biological prematurity in childhood. For a girl, this wait takes place in playful scenarios, such as playing with dolls. Girls mirror and dramatise all maternal cares by dressing, feeding, and talking to their dolls, reproducing playfully the maternal roles. Upon reaching puberty, the female body and its transformations acquire a trophic function, as Freud (1914, p. 88) points out:

> With the onset of puberty the maturing of the female sexual organs, which up till then have been in a condition of latency, seems to bring about an intensification of the original narcissism.

From a Freudian perspective, the desire for a child is the heir of the Oedipus complex and the pre-Oedipus in women, and it waits until puberty-adolescence to materialise. I see this as a waiting process for a future woman's body. In this path, many adolescents shift from childhood to motherhood without transition when they become pregnant—whether or not the pregnancy is carried to term.

Aulagnier distinguishes between the desire for a child and the desire for pregnancy. Following her ideas, the desire for a child is predominantly inscribed in the symbolic dimension and implies recognition of maternal castration. On the other hand, the desire for pregnancy is fundamentally related to the imaginary dimension in which the child is not predominantly perceived as an independent self, an object detached from the mother. The former concept concerns having a child, and the desire is the desire to have a child. It implies breaking with narcissistic alignment, renouncing the state of fusion and completeness. But in the case of the desire for pregnancy, the idea is to be with a child, who becomes part of the mother's libidinal economy. In this case, there is an illusory sense of unity with a demand to fuse in the mother-child bond.

We also know that there is always a temptation and a possibility that the child becomes part of a new illusion aimed at completing the woman. When we address the desire for a child within the clinical field, we may ask ourselves, along with Aulagnier (1992), What do I desire? From what child? as in the title of one of her works on this subject.

In the following pages, we address the concept of desire for a child from Freudian and post-Freudian perspectives, analysing similarities and differences.

Looking into Freud's theory

Freud's perspective on female sexuality was framed by different cultural variables, in which patriarchal supremacy was dominant and unquestioned. He was raised in an androcentric society, where women and men had quite specific and different roles allowing no discussion in the scientific field. Freud's contemporaries described women as incomplete beings (cited in Langer, 1951, p. 20). Initially, he studied the development of male sexuality and proposed an analogy for female sexuality, "As you see, I have only described the relation of a boy to his father and mother. Things happen in just the same way with little girls, with the necessary changes" (Freud, 1916–1917, p. 333).

This parallelism crumbles around 1920. In his article "The Infantile Genital Organization" (Freud, 1923b), he highlights the importance of phallic primacy and its central role for both genders. He acknowledges that "unfortunately we can describe this state of things only as it affects the male child; the corresponding processes in the little girl are not known to us" (p. 142). In 1925, Freud writes about the psychic consequences of the anatomic difference in young girls and its impact on the construction of the Oedipus complex: they become aware of the lack of a penis and therefore want to have one. Penis envy—like a narcissistic wound—may leave a scar related to a sense of inferiority.

At this point, he says that:

> The girl's libido slips into a new position along the line—there is no other way of putting it—of the equation 'penis-child'. *She gives up her wish for a penis and puts in place of it a wish for a child*[1]: and with that purpose in view she takes her father as a love object. Her mother becomes the object of her jealousy. The girl has turned into a little woman.
>
> (Freud, 1925, p. 256)

This paragraph has been quoted a million times to describe Freud's desire for a child in women as a replacement and removal of the desire for a penis. For a young girl to achieve her femininity, she is presented with a twofold change: the mother-father change—change of object—and the leading sexual organ change: from clitoris to vagina—change of erogenous zone. These modifications are based on acknowledging the anatomic differences between bodies and the meaning related to each difference.

The mother-father change is motivated by the young girl's penis envy. Later, it is the desire for a child that replaces the desire for a penis and takes control of feminine sexuality. At this point, Freud says that for the young girl, the Oedipus complex becomes a secondary construction, preceded by and built upon the reminiscences of the female castration complex. The main consequence of the young girl's discovery of the lack of a penis and the clitoris's "inferiority" is an increased tendency to feel inferior to men and to show jealousy about it.

According to Freud (1925), the Oedipus complex in girls is constructed by a superego, but with some distinct characteristics: it is less relentless, less impersonal, and less independent from its affective origins than in boys. He also adds that women show less sense of justice than men and are also less inclined to face life's great exigencies. They allow their tender or hostile feelings to lead them while making decisions. However, a boys' Oedipus complex construct implies a different superego. The Oedipus complex succumbs to the castration complex by identification with the father.

In 1917, Freud analyses the relations between a *child* and a *penis*, addressing the desire for a child in women, along with their anal equivalents. While researching female neurosis—one of the consequences of the relation between the desire for a child, and the desire for a penis in women with strong masculinity—he discovered that this pathology, together with an accidental failure, reactivates penis envy, which becomes the main reason for the presence of neurotic symptoms.

Other women do not show this desire for a penis, but instead a desire for a child, whose frustration can lead to the outbreak of a neurosis. Denied motherhood not only reactivates female castration complex anxiety but also increases the chances of suffering from neurosis. For Freud, this is the second location of the desire for a child and the desire for a penis in women. To expand this Freudian hypothesis, in the next chapter, we discuss a passion for a child, a maternal neurosis related to the frustration produced by the desire for a child. Lastly, Freud proposes a third case, in which both desires were present in women in childhood and relieved each other. First, they wished to have a penis from a man, and then they desired to have a child.

The female castration complex gives rise to the desire for a child, which appears first in the background. Initially, girls desire a penis like a boy's, which is then replaced—through a shift—by the desire for a child. It is a desire—as seen so far—related to genitality and the construction of the Oedipus complex. The desire for a child in girls is what leads them to desire a man, not the other way around: "and thus puts up with the man as an appendage to the penis" (Freud, 1917, p. 129).

From the point of view of object-choice, the love for the child is what "made [women] capable of an erotic life based on the masculine type of object-love, which can exist alongside the proper feminine one, derived from narcissism" (Freud, 1917, p. 29). Thus, the child—as a love object—is what allows the transition from narcissistic love to an object of love (Freud, 1914). Later on, Freud regrets the darkness surrounding the study of female sexuality. He even names it a dark continent: "We know less about the sexual life of little girls than of boys. But we need not feel ashamed of this distinction; after all, the sexual life of adult women is a 'dark continent' for psychology" (Freud, 1926, p. 212).

During the 1930s, Freud introduces significant modifications to his theories on female sexuality (Freud, 1931). For the first time, he analyses the pre-oedipal stage in girls and stresses the intensity and the extensive duration of this stage. He also describes the importance of this strong, initial affective bond. He focuses on a fundamental fact: both boys and girls aim their libidinal impulses towards the same object: the mother or her substitute. Boys love a woman from the very beginning, whilst girls detach from the mother and move towards the father (Freud, 1931).

He also highlights that father fixation in girls is nothing but the repetition of a previous mother fixation, with the exception that this initial bond remains throughout childhood. This bond is modified in the oedipal stage, when disappointment arises from the discovery of maternal castration, along with criticism that she made her "incomplete."

At this point, Freud says that girls must undergo three important changes in their libidinal structure: they must abandon the mother and target the father, send clitoridal excitability to the vagina, and turn their active sexual objectives into passive ones. Following these notions, we may assume that a girl's sexuality does not result in implicit heterosexuality, since it is the desire for a child that produces—through the girls' libidinal history—the desire for a man.

The desire for a child in a girl—from this perspective—is central, since it is immersed in the pre-oedipal bond with the mother. Identification with the mother works in two stages: in the pre-oedipal because girls take their mother as a role model and then in the positive Oedipus because they want to replace her and be with their father. That is why Freud insists that the pre-oedipal stage is crucial for a woman's future.

So far, we have analysed Freud's concept of desire for a child from the pre-oedipal and phallic perspectives. However, it is also related to the pre-genital organisation of the anal-erotic libido.

In 1917, Freud stated that:

> The baby is regarded as 'lumf' (…), as something which becomes detached from the body by passing through the bowel. A certain amount of libidinal cathexis which originally attached to the contents of the bowel can

thus be extended to the baby born through it. (...) the products of the unconscious—spontaneous ideas, phantasies and symptoms—the concepts faeces (money, gift), baby and penis are ill-distinguished from one another and are easily interchangeable.

(Freud, 1917, p. 130)

Part of the interest in faeces is split between the desire for money and the *desire for a child*. That is why the child is cathected with strong anal-erotic interest. The idea which social experience teaches us that a child is an act of love, a gift, is another concept that supports this pre-genital hypothesis. An analogy between faeces and penis is proposed, since the castration process represents the way in which the penis becomes an element that can be detached from the body.

Therefore, in the genesis of the desire for a child, we find a common point between an anal-erotic and a genital impulse. The latter derives from the Oedipus complex construction, linked to penis envy.

To summarise, we can say that Freud's perspective suggests the following hypotheses related to the desire for a child in women:

- The difference between men and women relies on anatomic differences and "the psychical situation involved in it" (Freud, 1925, p. 257).
- For young girls, the Oedipus complex forms in the background: they accept castration as a fact, whereas boys fear the possibility of it happening. Girls distance themselves from masculinity to allow their femininity to blossom.
- Freud says:

> Renunciation of the penis is not tolerated by the girl without some attempt at compensation. She slips—along the line of a symbolic equation, one might say—from the penis to a baby. Her Oedipus complex culminates in a desire, which is long retained, to receive a baby from her father as a gift—to bear him a child. (...) The two wishes—to possess a penis and a child—remain strongly cathected in the unconscious and help to prepare the female creature for her later sexual role.
>
> (Freud, 1924, p. 178)

- The desire for a child responds to a phallic instinct associated with the desire for a penis, which is referred to as *penis envy* when applied to women.
- The anal-erotic pre-genital libido is present in the desire for a child in the equivalence: penis-faeces-child.
- The desire for a child is related to the pre-oedipal stage in which girls take their mothers as a role model: to be a mother like their own.
- The desire for a child is what leads women to desire a man and not the other way around.

- Within this notion, we find two opposing libidinal concepts: on the one hand, a narcissistic libido—as a phallic equivalent—and, on the other hand, a change from narcissism to object-love.[2]

New perspectives: Post-Freudian authors

In 1920, different and fresh viewpoints regarding female sexuality arose in the psychoanalytic movement, which led to different ways in which questions emerge. The so-called *British movement*—whose main representatives include Ernest Jones, Karen Horney, and Melanie Klein—strengthens the idea of female nature and proposes a profound review of the Freudian hypothesis on primary masculinity in young girls—seen from a phallocentric perspective. Since then, there has not been any univocal view on the subject.

Jones—along with Klein—affirms the idea of a young girl's unconscious knowledge of the vagina. He proposes the existence of two sexes—departing from Freud's phallic monism—and that penis envy is not a primordial concept for a girl, but rather a defence mechanism (Jones, 1935). For Karen Horney, ignorance of the vagina stems from repression, and the girl's attachment to the clitoris acts as a defence mechanism.

Klein (1980) reformulates the notion of the way the psychic structure is organised: it is anxiety that moves and fuels the psyche. Human beings escape or defend themselves from this anxiety related to the death drive. Anxiety is the purest representation of the death drive. As opposed to Freud, who situates the Oedipus complex, as orbiting around object-love approximately at the age of 3, Melanie Klein's version of the Oedipus complex appears early on, although it is related to identification rather than to desire. If the girl identifies with her mother, the Oedipus is positive; if she identifies with the father, it is negative. This author—together with Ernest Jones and Karen Horney—as we said, hypothesises that girls have unconscious knowledge of the vagina.

Freud considers that there is only one sex. It is around it that the concept is built, with the polarity between two types: phallic or castrated. However, for Klein, there is the boy's sex and the girl's sex. Regarding libido, she again has a different point of view from Freud, who holds the notions of masculine libido and primary masculinity that girls go through during their first phase. Klein affirms that both sexes come from femininity and that masculinity in boys also derives from femininity. She supports this idea by arguing that the first love object for both sexes is the mother, and both identify with her.

In this way, Klein starts from an initial female position, as opposed to Freud's initial masculine position. She proposes that, with this identification, the girl has—according to oral logic—an impulse to bite things off of her mother, and fears being torn off and hurt by her. In Klein, the inside is more important than the outside. This means that the relationship with internal objects is more difficult than the relationship with external objects. These hypotheses allow us to draw some conclusions: the mother's inner body is a privileged scenario, in which both knowledge and conflict coexist. Here we find Klein's concept of babies: babies grow inside the mother's body and are equivalent to a child, penis, money, faeces, and breast.

As mentioned, she proposes an Oedipus complex that occurs earlier in terms of development than Freud's. It takes place during the first year of life and its development is different in girls and boys. Initially, the girl identifies with the mother, but at the same time, she must face a female castration complex related to feeling threatened of losing her internal body, or having it destroyed.

Regarding penis envy, again we find different perspectives in Freud and Klein. Freud considers that women enter the Oedipus complex castrated, which results in penis envy being central in women, and relegates the Oedipus complex to a secondary formation. However, Klein says that what is actually a secondary formation is penis envy, whereas what occupies a central role for women is primary castration anxiety, which is associated with fear of the destruction of their internal bodies.

Regarding the early Oedipus complex in girls, they identify first with the mother and desire to have the mother's babies inside of them, or to simply get the mother pregnant with their baby. When hatred for the mother appears, they identify with the father, with which a desire to have the father's penis to get the mother pregnant comes into play. At the same time, because of this hatred, they fear retaliation from their mother. Boys identify with the father and his penis.

In Klein—as already mentioned—the inside is much worse than the outside. But going back to female sexuality, this author proposes female maternal identification for both sexes as a starting point. She adds that the masculine perspective of women serves as a defence mechanism. Within this movement, and with the construction of the desire for a child, which derives from maternal identification, the girl faces a strict maternal superego, which Klein calls the bad mother.

In my view, this perspective provides new possibilities for the study of reproductive difficulties and their repercussions on women's psyche: ambivalence and hostile feelings towards the mother or other women, together with conscious or unconscious fantasies about having a damaged body. The different vicissitudes and conflicts concerning motherhood and obstacles to achieving it are described in clinical cases presented in this book.

Returning to Klein, her theory is radically different from Freud's. He says that girls desire a penis but, since they cannot have one, they compensate for this feeling by developing the desire for a child and aligning with the paternal figure. Klein argues that it is the other way around: the baby is the initial element, later replaced by the penis. In her child psychoanalysis studies, she mentions that the composition of the mother's inner body, as well as toys, becomes a privileged place of interest for children. It serves as the fuel to know about the mother's inner body and to develop the epistemophilic drive.

Maternity and its relation with the mother's body are central in Klein's theories.

To summarise, we can say that the *Viennese Movement* proposes the existence of primary masculinity in little girls, which derives from prejudice against penis envy in the female Oedipus. The *English Movement* proposes primary femininity and considers penis envy a secondary element in the construction of femininity, thereby strengthening the notion of a female character. The existence and place of the desire for a child within this framework also have theoretical-clinical implications on the way we conceive femininity and the place of everything female.

In the 1950s, Marie Langer (1951), in her book *Maternidad y Sexo* [*Maternity and Sexuality*], discusses women's conflicts and investigates the struggle between their professional work and maternal instincts. She points out that self-realisation for a woman was maternity and emphasises how culture influences each woman's life. She stresses that a woman can develop a full life and sublimate her maternal instinct. In later years, she criticises her previous ideas about the "natural desire to procreate" and the notion of "maternal instinct," shifting her initial essentialist perspective (Langer, 1982).

In *Maternity and Sexuality*, Langer (1951) discusses *reproductive disorders*—as she calls them—from a female sexuality perspective. She notes that key problems for women during Freud's time, framed by Victorian morality, were related to their repressed sexuality, which eventually caused frequent cases of hysteria. However, during the 20th century, when sexuality took a different place in culture, reproductive disorders become the main cause of conflict for women, with psychosomatic consequences. This is the way the conflict between maternity and sexuality arose.

These theories described by Marie Langer are clinical observables: the number of reproductive disorders has increased, as well as the abortion rate related to this disorder, while the mortality indicators that these abortions produce have not diminished. All these facts are true, despite the technological developments in reproductive medicine and oral contraceptive methods, which have been available since the sixties.

Freud's view on women's psychosexual development was also revisited by Marika Török (1964), who introduced a different perspective compared to the Freudian hypothesis of primary penis envy in women. This is an important contribution since primary penis envy is directly connected with the desire for a child in Freud's theory. Török stresses that penis envy in women is always the envy of an idealised penis. She points out that what is envied is not the attribute of the penis but the acts that make it possible to dominate things in general.

Tubert, in turn, analyses the desire for a child from the perspective of the French movement in her book *Mujeres sin sombra: maternidad y tecnología*

[*Women without a Shadow: Motherhood and Technology*] (1991). Following Lacan's perspective, she presents the phallus as a signifier of desire and decentralises it as an anatomic referent. She posits that the Oedipus complex has an inter-subjective structure, organised by free spots or positions that can be filled by different figures. They are not fixed values or self-defined spots; both are present and each exists because of the other: in Lacan, the Oedipus is the description of a structure and the effects its representation and subjectivation produce.

Lacan introduces a fourth element to the three figures within the Oedipus structure—father, mother, and child—the phallus, which supports the complex's articulation. The phallus represents something missing (Lacan, 1957–1958, as cited by Tubert). It is the element that stands for what it is missing and appears in its place. This author states that the imaginary phallus completes this missing spot and exacerbates a person's narcissism, since they feel that nothing is missing anymore (Lacan, 1957–1958, as cited by Tubert). Lacan's Oedipus complex consists of a binary opposition: to be or not to be the phallus, to have it or not. It is developed in three stages, which are determined based on the place the phallus occupies in the desires of each of the three main figures (Lacan, 1957–1958, as cited by Tubert). Any object can perform the phallus' imaginary function of filling this spot. Within female sexuality, the child's place and its symbolic equivalents have a central role. She points out that, when a woman says she wants to have a child, this expression does not unequivocally reference a real child. She discusses women's lack of awareness of desire. The desired object—the child—is desired in its symbolic function, not in its material form. Maternity is not just a privileged relationship between a woman and the real through the process of carrying a child in her body, it also places her as a mother inside a symbolic order.

Tubert stresses the importance of distinguishing desire from demand for a child. Demand for a child always refers to a demand to satisfy a need, in this case the child, but it is always a demand for love (Lacan, 1966). Need is placed within the biological, natural order of things, and desire is what impels a person to find absolute satisfaction: an impossible task.

Another psychoanalyst who has also developed her ideas about the desire for a child is Glocer Fiorini (2001). She develops the notion of desire for a child expanding the boundaries of the symbolic equation. Glocer Fiorini says that even though maternity has a natural root, it also thoroughly transcends it, locating itself within the realm of culture, a symbolic universe. Framed within the psychoanalytic conceptualisation that places maternity within a phallic logic, she highlights that the child emerges as a symbolic substitute derived from a fundamental sense of lack. She also wonders whether the substitutive nature of the desire for a child could be conceived in a different way.

She then proposes a notion of desire and considers that the child, as a product that causes desire, implies another conceptualisation of desire, detached from a philosophy of lack, which is a negative philosophy. According to her, desire should be conceived as a product that stimulates, which leads her to present the child as something more than just a substitute for a fundamental lack, opening the possibility for us to consider female subjectivity beyond maternity. In this perspective, the desire for a child transcends both the field of demand and the symbolic equation, becoming a project and a creation in a temporal dimension. Therefore, she presents differences between a child as a consequence of demand, a child as a phallic value—a product of the symbolic equation—and a child as a product that causes desire (Glocer Fiorini, 2001).

Tubert and Glocer Fiorini agree on this point when they differentiate the child as a result of demand from the child as a phallic value derived from the Freudian symbolic equation.

Acknowledging radical otherness in a child, Glocer Fiorini (2001) notes, allows the emergence of something original, the possibility of acknowledging something different, the creation of an experience beyond the borders of narcissism, and the possibility of exceeding the object relation. These ideas are related to a mother able to process her Oedipus complex, her grief, and the significance of a child.

In turn, Tajer (2013) poses a revision of the idea of the constitution of the desire for a child from gender theories. It is currently considered an imaginary effect of the relationship between motherhood and femininity historically constructed in modernity. These ideas allow us to think about motherhood within the desire and non-desire for a child, within the paradigm of complexity which gives rise to a plural desire, rather than a unique and hegemonic women's desire.

From a single to a plural desire

We can consider that there is one feature that has undoubtedly characterised women in psychoanalysis: a unique and hegemonic desire, the desire for a child. It is important to recall that the psychosexual development of girls is explained based on the primary masculinity seen in the desire for a penis, which later develops into penis envy.

Penis envy is a central theoretical concept and alludes to the absence, the wound, and the narcissistic affront of missing something essential. From this perspective, every woman desires to have and envies those with a penis. Girls enter the oedipal stage castrated, thus leading to the eventual desire for a child.

A girl's masculinity is based on the non-perception of her vagina, as stated by Freud, which was questioned a hundred years ago. The British School, as we said, deals with primary femininity for both sexes and the perception of the vagina in girls.

Finally, the desire for a child in the oedipal stage is defined by Freud (1925) by stating that the girl's libido slips into a new position along the line of the penis = child equation. The girl gives up her desire for a penis and puts in place of it a desire for a child.

Freud's use of the words "slips" and "equation" brings a linear and almost natural causality to his statement, especially in the idea of a pre-existing process in women.

In turn, the masculinisation of the girl when being envisaged as a boy is linked to the androcentric and patriarchal ideals that ruled at the time, with well-differentiated roles for men and women, which coexist to this day. Freudian vision of feminine sexuality was inevitably influenced by the cultural variables by which male supremacy was not questioned. In this regard, the questions that are raised are the questions that can be thought of in each epoch.

The desire for a child is in his work not only in the phallic stage as the resolution to the Oedipus complex but also in other theoretical axes such as the equivalence among child = penis = faeces = gift in anal erotism (Freud, 1917). In his paper *On Narcissism: An Introduction* (1914), the role of the child, described as "His majesty the baby," is associated with narcissistic parenting through desires projected onto the child to come and also through transcendence. In that same paper, Freud describes a type of narcissistic object in which the child is loved as part of the mother's body. Lastly, the desire for a child is also present in the girl's pre-oedipal stage in the identification of the girl with her mother's image: to be a mother like her mother (Freud, 1933).

There are several theoretical assumptions underlying Freudian developments about the desire for a child in women. Amongst them, we find phallic monism in how the girl is perceived as a boy, which also rests on binary logic. French anthropologist Françoise Héritier (1996) points out that the difference between the sexes contains a hierarchy within itself, one of them having pre-eminence over the other. She calls this *the differential valence of the sexes* within the difference between the sexes.

Lastly, an essentialist perspective is present in Freud's work in the fact that he defines women's journey into femininity through motherhood, meaning that motherhood makes the feminine being, in an ahistorical and immutable way.

If we think about how women's desire for a child is at the theoretical core of femininity, we can see the risk of clinical interpretation privileging motherhood as being intrinsic to femininity. This perspective naturalises the maternal in an unquestionable way, a vision that is underlain by the sacralisation of the maternal (Alkolombre, 2022).

Current scenarios are undergoing transformations regarding maternal-feminine and the notion of desire for a child. Facing possibilities ranging from the desire to have a child to the desire not to have a child, motherhood raises the necessity of deconstructing the classic paradigm of the feminine in the context of psychoanalysis. This paradigm is challenged by women's diverse experiences that do not adhere to the traditional conceptions of the feminine.

We can explore this issue by paraphrasing Freud's famous question to Marie Bonaparte: What do women want today when it comes to the desire for a child? It is a question that introduces us to a plural feminine, far from the idea that there is a unique destiny for femininity: the desire for a child as the result of the symbolic equation penis = child.

When we think about the notion of desire for a child, we can see the hegemony of maternity based on anatomical difference as biological support and, from the perspective of psychoanalysis, theoretical and traditional support. This means that when we discuss the desire for a child, we are thinking of the Oedipus complex in women and the correspondence between desire and penis envy.

From an essentialist and binary Freudian perspective, what women desire is defined by a unique path: maternity as a central part of their femininity. It maintains that there is a nature to femininity for all women, an understanding of maternity rooted in the sediment of patriarchal culture.

However, clinical experience shows us different scenarios in which diverse desires are present. Their voices in our consultation rooms are introducing us to new plural female experiences in the first person. We can also find the diversity of desires that unfold in new family configurations, many of them made possible by reproductive medicine.

In different clinical scenarios, we find women resorting to egg donation and women opting to become single mothers through anonymous insemination from a sperm bank, a growing practice. Other women become surrogates so others can become parents. Some maternities arise later in life; some women choose to preserve their fertility through ovum freezing, others decide to adopt children, and an increasing number of women choose not to have children at all. Some pregnancies are pursued against all odds, stemming from the passion for a child, which I develop in the following chapter.

Lastly, some women, for many reasons, decide to interrupt a pregnancy. We know from a clinical perspective the psychic consequences of the criminalisation of abortion: the scenarios of suffering and stigmatisation of women, adolescents, and girls. In many countries around the world, legislation prohibits abortions, especially in Latin America where I live and work.

In each expression of motherhood, fantasies and experiences are associated with the woman's unique history, which is determined by the socio-historical context and its practices. As already noted, all these alternatives have been made possible by advances in reproductive medicine unimaginable a few decades ago. We all know that the traditional ways of procreating—in the intimacy of sexual intercourse—exist since the beginning of humankind, whereas those initiated by medical-technological interventions were inaugurated in 1978.

We can say today that, whatever shape desires to have a child may take, motherhood challenges us to deconstruct the classic paradigm of maternal femininity in the light of psychoanalysis, together with the contributions of gender theories.

If we return to the question of what women want today when it comes to maternity, we find that there is much said by women about themselves. In our consulting rooms, we listen to their stories, their desires, and their suffering, whether or not they want to become mothers.

Historically, motherhood is associated with certain naturalisation of a desire considered typically feminine: the field of women's desire is almost entirely saturated with motherhood. It is important to revisit the different perspectives on the subject in the context of women's experiences of motherhood, ranging from the desire for a child to no desire at all. In this regard, today's maternities present the need for a decentralised interpretation of binarism and essentialism, within a desiring diversity. The maternal today is a heterogeneous territory encompassing changes in different family structures and gender identities.

Some notes on female infertility

Not long ago, when a couple[3] could not get pregnant, they were presented with two options: start the journey towards adoption or accept a life without children.

Nowadays, when they initiate the path to get a baby, they do not appear spontaneously but usually start by visiting the doctor. Women often visit their gynaecologist first and then a fertility specialist. During that process, they have to face two ideals: the infantile ideal of having a child "naturally" at a certain point in life and the ideal of control over their reproductive capacities, a concept present in society since the discovery of oral contraceptive methods.

As visits to the doctor become frequent, the body also moves gradually more and more to the centre of the stage: it is explored, analysed, and measured. The processes couples have to go through are tied to particular transient nature, since a peremptory feeling influences them. As time passes, the difficulties in getting pregnant and the presence of the hope-despair duality slowly permeate their daily lives.

This desire questions the body. The absence of a child becomes a pain, seen as such only when the desire to have a child and the impossibility to get one appear. Couples then start to experience a life marked by a single word: waiting.

We briefly explain these processes involving the desire for a child, the exposed body, and a special transitory state.

Within this context, we see how cultural heritage is responsible for introducing this central idea about maternity being an inherent realisation of femininity. In many cases, this concept leaves couples with reproductive disorders in a complicated situation.

For many women, the possibility of not having a child becomes a threatening idea. They enter a crisis that makes their life goals and identity as women falter. "Who am I, if not a mother?"

Without the pregnancy-baby combo, they are left without the necessary tools to achieve what should be a woman's destiny: to be a mother.

Both organic and psychic realms give us different ways to represent infertility. How do expectations and reality intertwine? Is what they are looking for inside the body? Or is it inside the mind?

One can anticipate a conflict between different roles and the role of the mother. Guite Guerin (1986) proposes that the relationship between a girl and her mother becomes a relationship between a woman and her own body. A body that cannot give birth to a child represents a mother denying that possibility to a woman. In this inner-psychic dynamic, it is no longer the mother who denies this woman the possibility of existing, but the body that denies the child that possibility. Guerin says that transforming into her own mother—who is related to her own body—is what grants a woman access to motherhood.

Infertility puts women back into a dual, specular situation, where the impossibility of being a mother is directly related to her own mother. Many patients trapped inside the pre-oedipal bond feel that there can only be a place for one mother: theirs. Without generational replacement, the transmission of psychic life is interrupted.

This conflict adds another reason to a girl's primary hate towards her mother for making her incomplete. First, she did not give her a penis during childhood, and now she denies her the possibility of getting pregnant, which deprives her of motherhood as well (Freud, 1931, 1933).

In the following sections, I develop ideas based on my clinical experience with patients searching for a child. Along this path, certain characteristics may be analysed more deeply: Fertile/infertile: a new symbolic equation?; The child's prehistory; A predictable body; and Temporality: living (through) the wait.

Fertile/infertile: A new symbolic equation?

Freud's perspective on female infertility can be considered a new version of a castration complex: in the absence of pregnancy, the oedipal conflict, which ended with the penis = child equation during childhood, reactivates and again confronts women with castration "embedded" in the body. It is not the lack of a penis, but the lack of a child.

This new version of the castration complex resignifies the phallic-castrated equation, which now becomes the fertile-infertile equation. For women—and men—their world has become a place defined by those who have children and those who do not. A clinical observable for this case is to see how all everyday activities are now framed in this idea: with friends, in family gatherings, work meetings, vacations, and birthdays. Everything is tainted by their lack of children since there are always "bellies" or children visible in these events.

There is pain and the experience of facing the fact of being different: not all the couples around them go through this problem. This particular fact produces persistent discomfort and, at the same time, an insistent question: Why do they have to carry this additional burden in life? Why are things not as easy as for others?

Reproductive difficulties evoke castration experiences since they impact the subject in its generative function. Silvia Vegetti Finzi (1990) considers that, in this situation, the subject faces, on the one hand, the fundamental oedipal prohibition: she says—referring to the impossibility of procreating a child—that you cannot be like your father and mother. But, on the other hand, the subject also faces an imperative command: you must be like your father and your mother—you must be father and mother.

The castration threat in infertility also references other signifiers and is translated into the Freudian expression: *narcissistic wound or injury*. Unconscious logic perceives the impossibility of carrying a child as a presupposed punishment. It is the expression of an act of castration. The impossibility of carrying a child highlights the desire for a child and imposes its presence.

The child's prehistory

In the first stages of a new life, we always find a previous story that allows us to look back and see the double dimension of an individual. Freud calls this *double existence*: to serve one's own purposes and to serve as a link in a generational chain (Freud, 1914). This particular fact provides the human life chain with a unique trait.

Michel Tort (1992) adds a characteristic when he affirms that there is no human reproduction since it is always marked by its symbolic significance. Reproduction, the process by which two individuals bring another one to life, is a symbolic operation that is socially organised in every culture.

Francoise Héritier (1992) says that not one single society considers birth only a biological process, since underlying this concept we find different systems of representation consisting of kinship, alliance, and filiation rules. These "agreed" representations ensure and strengthen the social bond and its existence and also give the child to be born an identification place: a framework for identifying references.

Reproduction derives from the term *re + produce*, from the Latin *prōdūcere* (Hoad, 2003). When we use the terms *reproduction* and *procreation*, we come across something extra, something new, a creation: a child.

From the point of view of anatomy, a pregnancy represents the mark of what is real in a woman's body, the point where the gametes meet to produce the fertilising act: ovum and spermatozoon. It is also the mark that represents the desired union for each member of the couple; a unique union, the support of conscious and unconscious psychic representations, blended in an instant.

Each child has a preceding story. Each father and mother has representations, desires, fears, and wishes about the child to come. It is the prehistory of the unborn child. Prehistory is marked by the way it is expected and by what its real existence will represent later in the unconscious of the parents and their projections.

For most women—from a psychic point of view—pregnancy carves into that long history that will then become the child's prehistory. Before conceiving, their psychic life is filled with fantasies about pregnancy: the child to be born and the mother she will become. These ideas are linked, at the same time, to the child they once were and to the mother they had. It is all about an imaginary child that will create dreams … or cause nightmares.

The imaginary child is "active" in a woman's mind before conceiving. Then, at birth, she will have to confront the real child, as proposed by Nerson-Sachs (1995).

In the clinical field of reproductive disorders, the time of the child-to-be-born's prehistory has different characteristics. It is prehistory that always includes medical records, a diagnostic search that "explains" the absence of pregnancy, medical studies and interventions, very long days and nights, menstrual blood, and tears. All these situations involve the body, trauma, and mourning.

For the couple, the child to be born is intensely cathected long before being conceived—sometimes even years before. Its birth also acquires different characteristics from those of a "naturally" produced pregnancy.

Reproductive difficulties impose a halt in the waiting stage, as well as a strong dependency on the group of ideas and affections surrounding the process of conception and the impossibility of making it happen.

A predictable body

When a couple starts seeking to have a child, pregnancy seems "natural"; it is only a matter of deciding to go ahead with it; the body will do the rest of the job. This natural characteristic is not only related to the biological processes involved but also to the idea of controlling the body's reproductive capacities. This idea has been supported by culture since the 1960s, with the appearance of oral contraceptive methods,[4] along with all the developments in reproductive medicine that emerged by the end of the 20th century: assisted fertility, a new method of human reproduction. Louise Brown, the first test-tube baby, was born in London in 1978.

As G says: "With pills I don't get pregnant, but if I stop taking them I will."

These scientific developments and their implementation have transformed the social imaginary and our knowledge of the body. David Le Breton (1990) does a profound analysis of the body's anthropology throughout history. He says that each society, within its inner vision of the world, creates a singular knowledge about the body, its functioning, its constituents, and its connections. The social framework, in this view, assigns value and meaning to the body.

Given all the improvements in reproductive medicine that occurred during the 20th century, Michel Tort (1992) proposes the idea of double inscription: one social and another made by each individual. He says that if we are to interpret the unconscious wagers proposed by the "new reproductive techniques," we should start with the proven fact that we are talking about a social phenomenon. It is not a small, individual fantasy, but a collective, endemic practice that, as symptomatic as it may seem, inserts two realities into the game: on the one hand, knowledge and scientific techniques, and on the other hand, sexual relations (Tort, 1992). Important questions are formulated in society to account for the collective and individual impact of these new devices.

From his perspective as a gynaecologist, Frydman (1986) proposes—following Tort's ideas—double inscription in these scientific developments. At the same time, he addresses some questions. He says that, as an individual, what one demands is apparently simple: a child. But collectively, something different is at stake, which explains the media's development of this subject. People are moved by surviving in a world in which nothing is a given. Solid notions such as life, death, father, and mother are disrupted. The constitutive schemes of their existence are dismembered. However, one should not underestimate the ideological crisis of the Western world. Unexpectedly, and thanks to medical science and biomedicine, fate will be defeated. People will be able to avoid the inexorable since fate is apparently more and more limited. The secrets nature is keeping will introduce new demands and new rights for people over her. But ultimately, he wonders if a right to a child exists.

Following these authors' ideas and their development, we may think that the current social imaginary proposes a body controlled by medicine and technology; what lies beneath these notions is the idea that everything is possible and that everything can be achieved. It is from this notion that a *predictable body* emerges as an imaginary product.

A *predictable body*[5] would be one we can foresee as having been modified by science and technique according to requirements and desires. As Frydman (1986) says ironically, a doctor would no longer ask a patient "what is hurting?" or "what is the matter?" but rather "what do you desire?"

In this way, the "old" infantile omnipotence is projected in today's science and techniques: the omnipotence the child attributes to their parents and the one children attribute to themselves. One may wonder about the difference between the idea of people using science to aid their health and well-being compared to the idea that people can be subordinated to serve science and technique by lending their body, their humanity, as if it were a "machine to be repaired." As M says: "If I don't get pregnant, I'll do *in vitro* fertilisation."

A *predictable body* anticipates the change a person is seeking by using a specific intervention on the body. The individual is decentralised since it is the technique that is responsible for the desired change.

The risk is that the individual may be "left aside," dissociated from the process of change. Many patients who undergo assisted fertilisation treatments cannot develop and integrate the transformations produced by medical-technological interventions. This may happen at any point in the different stages of the process: during diagnosis or treatment, especially in all treatments in which technology plays a crucial role: assisted fertilisation, processes of ovum donation (OD) or sperm donation (SD), pre-implantation genetic diagnosis,[6] to mention a few.

In this way, the person's known and familiar body can become something unknown: a human duplicate, something *unheimlich* or uncanny (Freud, 1919).

Against this idea perceived by part of the social imaginary that nowadays we are in the presence of a *predictable body*, psychoanalytic clinical work shows that desires pulsate from the unconscious, live in all individuals, and remain with them forever. These desires also reveal that we are vessels of an "unpredictable" body. The peculiar geography analysed by Freud in "the hysterias," during the early days of psychoanalysis, accounts for the body's polysemic language.

Temporality: Living (through) the wait

Working out infertility can take a lot of time. It is the impasse of a body, a frozen image, a timeless present. It is a signifier that entails a sense of emptiness, of time wasted, of time lost.

Different times may be distinguished. The time required for medical studies and the time needed to consider sterility in some way: accepting it, figuring it out, or envisaging an adoption. This time makes it possible to stop having a non-sense, a no-place. It enables the acquisition of an endurable, acceptable sense.

L says, "I wanted to have a child to forget my mother."

The only pleasant expectation of waiting times involved in infertility treatments is the possibility of pregnancy, which is the only source of anticipated pleasure. The image of pregnancy projects itself throughout menstrual cycles, as if on a screen.

The gap between sexual activity and reproduction in couples begins to open, leading to an increase in sexual desire during the peak of ovulation:

a possible encounter between the bodies in the fertile period, which then decreases. It may be in this cycle, the next ovulation, or the next treatment.

Time and the body's ups and downs are adjusted in a clockwork that cannot be synchronised. Pleasure and desire become duty and desire. The search becomes in itself a long pregnancy, and a phenomenon takes place, similar to the one described by Freud (1916) in his article on the transitory: sorrow for something unattainable leaves the couple suffering and with a sense of loss. Like the poet who suffered about the transience of the beauty of flowers, as time passes in spite of her *biological clock*, women in particular begin to feel the same state of anticipated loss.

This observation goes beyond the implementation of techniques that compensate for the effects of time. Such is the case of maternity in menopausal women. In these situations, the ageing of gametes is overcome through the donation of young women's ova. This is also true when organic issues are involved, such as in women with primary ovarian insufficiency.[7] For these women unable to procreate with their own ova, the choices are adoption, a childless life, or resorting to OD.

In these processes, temporality is different in men because they biologically produce spermatozoa throughout their lives. This is permanent since puberty. Their view of the horizon is not as clearly defined as it is for women. They have no experience comparable to a biological clock.

The fruitless search for pregnancy very often leads women to a dead end where the child becomes the only chance for a future. Every interest, relationship, and activity developed is de-cathected. Following the hypothesis raised by Freud (1914) in "On Narcissism: An Introduction," women's pre-occupation with the way their body works makes their libido withdraw and then cathect reproductive capacity.

It is universally known, and we take it as a matter of course, that a person who is tormented by organic pain and discomfort gives up his interest in the things of the external world, in so far as they do not concern his suffering (Freud, 1914, p. 82).

This description suggests an alteration in the distribution of libido: a withdrawal into itself, narcissistic confinement. Patients live [through] the expectation of a pregnancy-baby. This restraint not only deprives them of possibilities but also deprives them of all the responsibility for the awareness of choice. Many patients start by giving up their activities one by one. This change is met with a certain social consensus: they are devoting themselves to "getting pregnant."

In this same line of thinking, Nancy Chodorow (1984), in *The Reproduction of Mothering*, remarks that the experience of pregnancy and the anticipation of motherhood entail, for many patients, abandoning any primary interest beyond their own bodies.

Living [through] the expectation in this manner defines a psychic space that leaves all other activities and interests in abeyance. Life goes on while they wait for the most important thing to arrive: a child. Everything this absence involves, especially others' babies and children, only exacerbates this waiting period.

So far, we have studied different theoretical perspectives regarding the multiple desires for a child in women. We will continue in the next section with a closer look at the desire for a child in men.

About men's desire

Our discussion of the desire for a child in men needs to be framed within conceptions of male sexuality. For a long time, the notion of desire for a child was conceived only from women's perspective, as evidenced by the emphasis placed on the mother-child rather than the father-child in psycho-analytic conceptualisations.

Throughout history, masculinity has suffered from the *taken-for-granted* syndrome—as Gilmore (1999) points out—mainly because of the abundance of literature about femininity. Although femininity and masculinity present their own specific issues, the masculine aspects generally tend to be implicit. In different cultures, men have to undergo certain ordeals and rituals to access masculinity. That is why—again, as Gilmore poses—men are not born as such, but rather have to *become men*.

The masculinity and virility picture has left other aspects of male sexuality out of the discussion. As mentioned before, the desire for a child belongs almost exclusively to the feminine realm, and this fact has caused conflict for men related to this generalised ideal of masculinity, presented culturally and associated with power, virility, and their role as providers.

The acquisition of a masculine identity starts with a process of identification, the earliest manifestation of an affective bond with parents and male social ideals. Gender perspectives present it as a nuclear gender identity, a child's perception that he is a boy since he is born.

The boy wants to be like his father and to replace him in everything; he is his role model. Thereby identifying with the father, he takes his mother as an object of desire. These notions coexist until the threat of castration appears. André Green writes that this threat is sometimes preceded, as was formerly common, by a threat verbalised by the mother or one of her substitutes (a nanny or a governess) to intimidate the boy and prompt him to give up auto-erotic pleasure. Even though women issued the threat, men were responsible for executing the consequences of crossing the line: the father, the doctor, etc. For the child, the realisation of the difference between sexes happens at the precise moment when they discover the presence of the penis (in boys) or its lack (in girls). When the Oedipus complex materialises, the threat of castration, at first denied or challenged, becomes psychically effective based on childhood sexual theory, since the boy fears being punished by castration (Green, 1992). Therefore, anxiety derived from masculine castration is firmly rooted in the Oedipus complex, particularly in the act of giving up his incestuous childhood love in favour of his narcissistic interest in preserving his penis.

In his article "Analysis Terminable and Interminable," Freud (1937) locates masculinity on the end of the activity, masculine = active, leaving passivity on the feminine-castrated end: "In males, the striving to be masculine is completely ego-syntonic from the first; the passive attitude, since it presupposes an acceptance of castration, is energetically repressed, and often its presence is only indicated by excessive overcompensations" (p. 230).

In all Freud-related theories, everything associated with femininity in men is considered a phantasy to become feminine. Boys firmly reject everything related to the feminine function of carrying a child in order to keep their masculinity unaltered, since they associate femininity with castration.

The castration complex in boys presents fantasies associated with the anus and the act of giving birth. André Green, referring to the story of little Hans and concerning this subject, states that the interest supporting Hans's ideas consists of showing that all concerns regarding castration are also connected to the act of defecation and the sexual theory related to giving birth. It is impossible to conceive of men's loss of virility without addressing the femininity conflict that affects them (Green, 1992).

Although in Freud's works there are no direct references to the desire for a child in men, this search takes us to the realm of fatherhood, which is related to boys' Oedipus complex history and prehistory.

The father's role is crucial to resolving the Oedipus complex. Initially, Freud proposed the Oedipus complex in connection with boys, later extending it to girls as well.

In the "simple" Oedipus complex, the girl falls in love with her father, the boy with his mother, and oedipal rivalry appears. Later on, Freud (1923b) presents the Oedipus complex notion, taking into account the affectionate desires of both parents, including both heterosexual and homosexual dimensions of desire: the positive and the negative Oedipus complex. Green (1992) describes the overall complex as consisting of two aspects: a positive or heterosexual one, a negative or homosexual one, and the joint strength of both elements. In general, both negative and positive aspects are "destroyed" by repression.

He proposes to define the Oedipus complex as the double-difference complex since it groups the fluctuating differences of both sexes and the differences between generations. The incestuous nature of infantile sexuality is repressed by severe prohibitions: the prohibition of incest and parricide in oedipal times.

The inverted or passive Oedipus complex represents a desire for sexual union with the parent of the same sex and the development of rivalry with the other parent. At this point, the boy must solve a conflictive situation: in this positive Oedipus complex, his incestuous sexual desires for his mother, he has to confront the threat of castration, while at the same time, in the negative Oedipus complex, his incestuous sexual desires for his father, he confronts the fact of being castrated. This conflict results in the creation of a new psychic agency: the superego, which enables the individual to enter the culture.

Mauricio Abadi (1960) addresses this problematic fatherhood, proposing a basic triangular oedipal relationship, mother, father, and child, that results from the intertwining between the generational conflict and the battle of the sexes.

Abadi stresses the importance of men's envy of women for their motherly and reproductive abilities, which as opposed to men represents a guarantee of an afterlife for women that counters death anxiety.

He considers that this envy drives men to fantasies about stealing the child and bonding with it. Abadi aims to identify more with the pregnant mother than with the procreating mother. This pregnant mother who wants to keep the child as part of herself has what he calls the *everlasting pregnancy fantasy*. This everlasting pregnancy phantasy is represented by the pregnant woman and, ultimately, by the man in *couvade* (Abadi, 1984). Abadi focuses on death anxiety, saying that the most important thing about life is its inescapable race towards death. The most *biological* defence mechanism developed by men to try to cope with death anxiety is procreation: to perpetuate oneself through a child, an exclusively feminine realm. This is what causes men's frustration for not being able to be a "mother."

Arminda Aberastury (1984) says that the subject of fatherhood was omitted in Freud's work and only developed after the appearance of child psychoanalysis. She highlights that Freud, while constructing the Oedipus complex, inconsistently twisted Sophocles' narration of the Oedipus myth. She states that he only considered the child's situation against the parents and did not address, or repressed, how the parents feel and act in relation to their children.

She wonders why Freud did not mention that Laius was the one who had sent the order to kill Oedipus, instead stressing that Oedipus killed Laius without knowing he was killing his father.

According to Aberastury, the explanation for this decision lies in Freud's Oedipus complex, in his decision not to judge Laius and consequently placing all the blame on Oedipus. The discovery of the Oedipus complex, the nuclear complex of neurosis, occurs in 1897 while Freud was working through his father's death by means of his self-analysis. At this time, he writes that the father's death is one of the most important moments in a man's life.

Aberastury also proposes the idea of men's desire to carry a child, a common desire in the first stages of a boy's development. She says that it is a homosexual period in which the boy desires to have relations with his father, take his mother's place, and have children.

This deep-rooted desire for a child affects men's repressive thoughts since homosexuality acts as its source. Aberastury's analysis of men's desire for a child takes into account the boy's affective impulses towards his father. These impulses and desires are repressed in two ways: from the inside and by the external world. She argues that boys, during their general developmental process, go from the desire to be inseminated by the father's penis to the desire and need to penetrate and inseminate the mother. On the other hand, the external world demands them to assume roles that mark their sexual differences from women. This means that both internal and external worlds force boys to repress their homosexual tendencies. Together with these, they also repress their desire for a child, which then becomes a forbidden subject, since it is a concept that implies carrying a child in their bodies. In conclusion, she says that, since childhood, the maternal origin of a father's role turns all fatherly feelings into something disturbing (Aberastury and Salas, 1984).

For the construction of the desire for a child in boys, she takes into account not only internal aspects related to the subject but also social determinants related to masculinity.

Nancy Chodorow (1984) articulates psychoanalytic and gender theories to propose the differentiated way of raising boys and girls: girls are raised for motherhood, whereas boys are soon removed from all domestic activities.

Another aspect that Aberastury mentions is boys' repression of the negative Oedipus complex and everything related to it: the desire for a child's "maternal" or "feminine" origin, since it implies the desire to have a child from the father, something that upsets men's role as fathers.

In many of his writings, Freud rejects femininity in men. For example, in "Draft M" he says:

> It is to be suspected that the essentially element repressed is always what is feminine. This is confirmed by the fact that women, as well as men, admit more easily to experiences with women than with men.
>
> (Freud, 1897, p. 251)

The same ideas are mentioned again in one of his last works, "Analysis Terminable and Interminable" (1937). There he introduces the concept of *bedrock*—penis envy in women—and the concept of *repudiation of femininity*, associated with men.

We may therefore consider that the desire for a child in men, when it involves a feminine perspective, is rejected since there is a confrontation, following Freud's ideas, between this concept and the bedrock or what is called the feminine (Freud, 1937). Fear of all passive and feminine things is quite intense since they are reminiscent of men's most powerful and repressed desires. Anything related to women, as castration presupposes, is rejected along with the desire for a child.

This perspective has been reviewed over time, confronting the idea that all feminine-related aspects in men are tied to their negative Oedipus, that is to say, their unconscious homosexual aspects, and that these aspects are not taken into account as part of their masculinity.

In turn, Groddeck (1923) observes that it is not uncommon to find somatic disorders in men related to concerns, generally unconscious, about a desire for, fear of, or an imaginary pregnancy in men. He wrote in a letter to a friend that she would scold him because he was again making merry over mothers. He continued that perhaps in part it was because of envy that he made fun of mothers, envy that he was not himself a woman and could not be a mother. He would ask her not to laugh at that for it was true, and true not of him alone, but of all men, even of those who seem most manly. Groddeck (1923) says that men's talk tells us that even the most masculine of men feels no hesitation in telling us that he is pregnant with some thought, refers to his brainchild, and speaks of the fulfilling of some laborious task as "a difficult birthing." And these are not just turns of speech. Groddeck told his friend that from her own memories of him, she would know that in some instances his stomach would swell up, but then if he spoke to her about it, it would suddenly subside. His friend knew, too, that he referred to this as "his pregnancy."

For Groddeck (1923), stomach aches, headaches, toothaches, nosebleeds, and vomiting are all symptoms that can be related to ideas of childbirth intertwined with sexual theories of children about conceiving and giving birth: anal and digestive theories.

Nasio (1991), in his article "La femineidad del padre" [The father's femininity], proposes that everyone who takes the father's place must acknowledge his feminine side. He also says that all men who painfully acknowledge their feminine sides have more chances of assuming the difficult role of being a father than those who do not acknowledge their femininity. For a neurotic, *his* femininity is a synonym of passivity and submission. For a man, being a woman means experiencing what the woman in his nightmare experiences. What does she experience? He concludes that what she experiences is the suffering of being castrated. A neurotically dreamt woman is indeed a castrated being, exposed and subdued to the perverse actions of an Other.

Nasio (1991) also stresses that, for men, the term *repudiation of femininity* means to reject it based on fear and an imaginary risk of losing a part of himself or even everything by the act of being subdued or dependent on another, capable of destroying him. However, he proposes that men who can accept their feminine side are those who were able to overcome all these sources of anxiety and were also able to understand that we always lose something and that it is inevitable.

In his interesting article *The Facts of Fatherhood* (1992), Thomas Laqueur takes into account what he calls the *emotional work* in fatherhood. At the beginning of the article, he regrets that there is no history of fatherhood because, throughout history, all knowledge related to being a man or a father was always silenced.

An article by Phyllis Chesler (1991) dedicated to mothers inspired Laqueur's article. Chesler explains that motherhood is "a fact," an ontological category different from fatherhood, which is considered "an idea."

Based on that premise, Laqueur narrates his experience as a father when his newborn daughter spent some time in a hospital in an incubator. He observed that, when his wife went to see her at the hospital, the staff wrote in the medical records: "Mother bonding." But when he was the one visiting, they wrote something affectively neutral: "Father's visit."

He proposes that facts about motherhood and fatherhood are not fixed. On the contrary, the relation between facts and their meaning is crucial.

In the same direction, Elisabeth Badinter (1993) states that the maternal instinct hypothesis supports the idea that the mother is the one who can take care of the child since, in her own words, she is biologically configured to do so. That is how mother-child pairing becomes an ideal unit, legitimising the father's exclusion and strengthening mother-child symbiosis. In her book *La part du père* (1981), Geneviève Delaisi de Parseval proposes the possibility of bringing the father's process of becoming a father to light.

There is still a long way to go in the field of the desire for a child in men, a terrain most certainly different from the desire for a child in women.

A new dark continent: Male infertility

The problem of male infertility deserves a separate book. Everything in relation to a man's place in consultations on infertility deserves to be studied. Much has been said and written about females and the problems affecting women in that field. In the literature, as well as in medical and psychoanalytic investigations, both the desire for motherhood and also the psychic repercussions in women in cases of infertility have been favoured.

The problem of men with reproductive difficulties and their desire for fatherhood has raised little interest or enthusiasm. Only recently, in the last few decades, scientists have acknowledged that, from the medical perspective, sterility in a couple is due to both the man and the woman (Perco, personal communication, 2008). Some decades ago, marital infertility was thought to have mainly a female origin. This gave women an exclusive place in consultations and little attention has been given to men. What is the place of the masculine in infertility? What phenomena have made something clinically observable invisible? (Alkolombre, 2017).

Historically, all that is related to parenthood has focused on women, leaving a man's desire for a child unexplored, under a veil of shadow.

Freud's Schreber case (Freud, 1911) is one of the few, along with the case of the Rat Man (Freud, 1909a), in which he mentions conjugal infertility.

In the former, Freud mentions the fact that Schreber had no children; this failed fatherhood, mostly due to the patient's complex relationship with his father, is not regarded as one of the root causes of the disease. Essentially, Freud attributed his pathology to his homosexual delusions.

Dr. Schreber had been ill twice. The first time was in 1884 when he expressed himself as follows:

> After my recovery from my first illness, I spent eight years with my wife - years, upon the whole, of great happiness, rich in outward honours, and only clouded from time to time by the oft-repeated disappointment of our hope that we might be blessed with children.
>
> (Freud, 1913, p. 12)

In another part of the record, Freud writes a note where he establishes a connection between the patient's delusion of becoming a woman and his inability to have offspring:

> Dr. Schreber may have formed a phantasy that if he were a woman he would manage the business of having children more successfully; and he may thus have found his way back into the feminine attitude towards his father that he had exhibited in the earliest years of his childhood.
>
> (Freud, 1913, p. 58)

Additional information about his life, published in the book *The Schreber Case* (Baumeyer, 1956), points out that his wife had six pregnancies that failed due to miscarriages and stillborn children. This fact was reported by his foster daughter. He also notes that, following his brother's death, Schreber was the only son left in his family.

In the text on Psycho-Analysis and Telepathy, Freud refers again to male sterility when he describes the case of a woman who was about to have gynaecological surgery until her husband talked her out of it. He "confessed" that it was he who could not have children:

> Only one thing was wanting: she was childless. She was now 27 years old and in the eighth year of her marriage. She lived in Germany, and after overcoming every kind of hesitation she went for a consultation with a German gynaecologist. With the usual thoughtlessness of a specialist, he assured her of recovery if she underwent a small operation. She agreed, and on the eve of the operation discussed the matter with her husband. It was the hour of twilight and she was about to turn on the lights when her husband asked her not to: he had something to say to her and he would prefer to be in darkness. He told her to countermand the operation, as the blame for their childlessness was his.
>
> (Freud, 1941 [1921], p. 186)

Here again, as in Schreber's records, there is no connection between patients falling ill and marital infertility. In the latter case, there is a direct reference to the shame the patient's husband feels when he has to "confess" this secret to her. We see how male sterility continues to be silenced and is experienced with shame. The latter is a feeling that manifests itself in intersubjectivity. It implies that someone else discovers something that undermines the individual.

In Freud's quotation, the patient's husband prefers darkness in which to tell her his secret, unspeakable in the light. We may think of the darkness that shrouds the topic of male infertility, the shame, and the ideas about the desire for a child in men that underlie these male feelings. I refer to this darkness in two works (Alkolombre, 2004, 2001), where I propose the idea of a *dark continent* to reflect on male infertility and the questions it involves: a dark area, under-researched: infertility as experienced by the male.

We know that stress has traditionally been placed on the man's social and economic role, as well as in his role as a genitor and the mother's companion. Men also hold the law in their hands. These androcentric traits are attributed to them: physical strength, success, money, and work. These ideas still dominate well into the 21st century.

Elizabeth Badinter (1993) undertakes a critical review of masculinity in her book *XY: On Masculine Identity*. She argues that the *myth of masculinity* survives thanks to the complicity of those who are oppressed by it. The drawbacks of the masculine archetype are even greater since many men are still far from reaching the mythical standard of success, power, self-restraint, and strength. The promotion of such an unattainable image of virility creates a painful awareness: the feeling of being incomplete as a man. Many men view hyper-masculinity as a remedy against that permanent insecurity, which leads them to become prisoners of obsessional, compulsive masculinity that not only makes their life impossible but also comes to constitute a source of self-destruction and aggressiveness against anyone who threatens to unmask them.

Virility, sexual potency, and fertility are equations associated with the male figure in the traditional social imaginary. Since these are all "narcissised" male functions, a man faced with losing the procreative function feels that part of his masculine identity is threatened.

Identity is a feeling that provides a sense of existential continuity, which is why individuals recognise themselves and are recognised by others despite changes. Throughout life, some crises bring about changes, some of them threatening identifications on which identity is founded. In the case we are considering, and based on the aforementioned clinical and medical records presented by Freud, we point out that the inability of men to have children has an impact. They need to work through mourning in a social context that dismisses men's desire for a child.

Our culture is devoid of representations of male infertility. The lack of a social network in these cases is clinically observable and the suffering involved remains hidden.

Considering that the first inseminations using donor sperm date back two centuries (Frydman, 1986), what is not being said? Perhaps it is men's suffering for being unable to have children: the impossibility of procreation.

What is the place of men in reproduction, according to their culture?

It is in their presence through the couvade, a phenomenon described by anthropologists as a ritual in which the man takes the place of the woman during labour. For the father, it is a way to join his child's birth. There is also the concept of a *natural child*, with no known father, and of the *bastard*, a fatherless child.

Men's role in reproduction presents itself as vicarious since they take someone else's place. It would seem that the man in reproduction occupies a place that may remain vacant, as suggested by the phrase *"pater semper incertus est,"* whereas the mother is *"certissima"* (Freud, 1909b, p. 1989).[8] Therefore, masculinity is more related to their ability to procreate.

In this line of thinking, Jacques Hassoun (1998) writes about virility. It seems that it has always been a matter of concern among men, for whom virility, as well as the ability to procreate, though not the ability to be a father, is part of their essence.

Working with men with reproductive disorders reflects the pain of facing a change in the dual destiny of the human being: to serve their individual purpose and to be a link in the generational chain (Freud, 1914).

Infertility impacts ideals associated with masculine identity and leads men to experience a rupture of the generational chain. It reveals the importance of blood ties and the need of affiliation for a sense of belonging: to be someone's child and someone's father. The absence of children is observed in both the Rat Man's case and Schreber's.

Based on Piera Aulagnier's (2003) concept of the narcissistic contract, the man identifies himself with the values of his culture to build his identity; in turn, society gives something back and embraces him, giving him a place where he belongs. Male infertility has no citizenship papers, and therefore it languishes in no man's land. In this sense, it is a dark continent. It has no referents in our society since we think about it in feminine terms.

It is often experienced in silence, painfully, as a traumatic situation, a withdrawal of support. In some cases, the experience of being "unmanly" may explain the tendency to resort quickly to sperm banks in order to end the situation.

Even though each man may overcome his difficulties, according to his characteristics and history, reflections are related to the possibilities and obstacles in the proceedings of this particular matter. It produces a destabilisation of the self-image, directly affecting narcissism. It may be experienced as a punishment, the enactment of the threat of castration. The latter would not be a loss of the penis, but the lack of spermatozoa, an "empty-ing" of the penis. The penis is under-cathected, whereas fertility becomes hyper-cathected.

Castration separates the sex organs from the body. However, strictly speaking, it consists of the deprivation of the means of reproduction. From this perspective, male infertility actualises castration anxiety. The man may face more primitive anxieties, influenced by the Oedipus complex dur-ing childhood when he had to give up incestuous love in exchange for his narcissistic interest in keeping his penis.

The threat of castration revived by the experience of infertility creates a reactivation of castration anxiety and, by displacement, is responsible for various symptoms observable in clinical practice: impotence, medical procedures, and various organic symptoms.

In this case, paraphrasing Freud, the psychic consequences of the differ-ence in sexual anatomy have different effects. What is not fertile, not potent, is strongly rejected. If a man does not have that valuable asset, does he come dangerously close to femininity, with the consequent fear of passivity or lack of virility? How do we make a place for grieving? At the same time, how do we think about the man's desire for a child?

Alienating the fertile-masculine and rejecting the castrated-feminine, a man's place in relation to the chance of having children is very often at a difficult crossroads.

Notes

1 Italics are mine.
2 During the sphincter control stage, children are presented with the first oppo-sition between narcissistic libido and object-love: they must decide between expelling and "surrendering" their excrement as an act of love or keeping it for their own erotic pleasure to reaffirm their personal power.
3 In this section, even though we are considering female infertility in a hetero-sexual couple as an object of analysis, it can also be thought of in the context of female single parenthood and sexual and gender diversity.
4 Contraception is a subject closely related to the beginning of psychoanalysis. Freud (1893) believed that the aetiology of neurasthenia was related to the contraceptive methods' harmfulness. He refers specifically to *coitus interrup-tus*, *condom intolerance*, and *extra-vaginal intercourse*, all used during married life with a view to preventing pregnancy. However, at the same time, they are all causes of neurasthenia, according to the toxic theory of neurosis.
5 It may be possible to extend the concept of the *predictable body* to other fields: genetic engineering, transplants, sex change surgery, life extension, plastic surgery, etc.
6 Ovum donation (OD): it is a therapeutic resource that consists of replacing the female gamete (ovum) with ova from a donor. It is prescribed for: steril-ity caused by premature ovarian failure, bad quality ova, repeated implanta-tion failure, bad quality embryo, sterility without apparent cause, inherited disease, and pre- and post-menopause. Sperm donation (SD): as in OD, the masculine gamete (spermatozoa) is replaced with sperms from a donor. It is

prescribed for: sterility caused by irreversible azoospermia, very bad sperm quality, and severe sperm DNA fragmentation. Pre-implantation genetic diagnosis (PGD): it is a state-of-the-art resource in which some genetic structures can be recognised in the embryo before being transferred to the body. It enables the recognition of certain embryo pathologies, as well as the sexual structure (XX or XY) and aneuploidy. The technique consists of removing an embryonic blastomere (cell) by micro-manipulation before the embryo is transferred to the uterus. The only embryos transferred are those free from any detectable genetic pathology (Perco, personal communication, 2008).

7 Primary ovarian insufficiency (POF): it is the premature failure of ovarian function (cessation of ovulation and estrogenic hormone production) before the age of 40. Initially, it is characterised by the absence of menstruation. Later, it shows symptoms similar to menopause (Perco, personal communication, 2008).

8 '"*Pater semper incertus est*," while the mother is '*certissima*"' is an expression used by Freud to analyse the phantasy in the neurotic's family romance. There he stresses the contrast between the uncertainty of biological fatherhood and the certainty of motherhood. In the neurotic's family romance, the boy imagines and creates a story in which he is the son of an idealised father (Freud, 1909, p. 1989). Nowadays, with the implementation of DNA analysis, it is possible to ascertain the father's genetics.

References

Abadi, M. (1960). *Renacimiento de Edipo: la vida del hombre en la dialéctica del adentro y del afuera* [*Rebirth of Oedipus: Man's Life in the Dialectic between Inside and Outside*]. Buenos Aires: Nova.

Abadi, M. (1984). El significado inconsciente del rol paterno: meditación sobre Layo [The unconscious meaning of the paternal role: meditation on Laius]. *Revista de Psicoanálisis, 33*(1), 121–148.

Aberastury, A., & Salas, E. (1978). La paternidad. In *La paternidad* (pp. 113–126), Buenos Aires: Kargieman.

Alkolombre, P., & Segundas Jornadas de Infertilidad, Adopción y Fertilisación Asistida APdeBA (2001). Esterilidad masculina, 'un continente negro?' [Male sterility—A dark continent?]. In Ed *Segundas Jornadas de Infertilidad, Adopción y Fertilización Asistida APdeBA,* Fertilización Asistida. Nuevos Avances, Nuevas Problemáticas (pp. 11–15). Buenos Aires: APdeBA.

Alkolombre, P. (2004). "Psicoanálisis y relaciones de género en fertilidad asistida" [Psychoanalysis and gender relations in assisted fertility]. In Alizade, M. & Lartigue, T. *Psicoanálisis y Relaciones de Género [Psychoanalysis and Gender Relations]* (pp. 79–91). Buenos Aires: Lumen.

Alkolombre, P. (2017). Vicissitudes of the desire to have a child in contemporary parenthood: Reproductive techniques and the new origins. In Holovko, C. & Thompson-Salo, F. *Changing Sexualities and Parental Functions in the Twenty-First Century* (pp. 87–101). London: Karnac.

Alkolombre, P. (2022) The maternal-feminine: Scenarios in transformation psychoanalysis and gender perspectives. In Cereijido, M.; Ellman, P.; Goodman, N., *Psychoanalytic Explorations of What Women Want Today* (pp. 161–171). London: Routledge.

Aulagnier, P. (1992). 'Qué deseo, de qué hijo?' [What desire? For what child?]. *Revista de Psicoanálisis con Niños y Adolescentes*, 3, 45–49.

Aulagnier, P. (2003). *La violencia de la interpretación* [*The Violence of Interpretation*]. Buenos Aires: Amorrortu.

Badinter, E. (1993). *XY, La identidad masculina* [*XY: On Masculine Identity*]. Colombia: Editorial Norma.

Baumeyer, F. (1956). The Schreber case. *International Journal of Psycho-Analysis*, *37*, 61–74.

Chesler, P. (1991). Mothers on trial: *The custodial vulnerability of women*. *Feminism & Psychology*, 1(3), 409–425.

Chodorow, N. (1984). *El ejercio de la maternidad. Psicoanálisis y sociología de la maternidad y paternidad* [*The Reproduction of Mothering: Psychoanalysis and the Sociology of Gender*]. España: Gedisa.

Delaisi de Parseval, G. (1981). *La part du père* [*The Father's Share*]. Paris: Editions du Seuil.

Ferenczi, S. (1988). *Diario Clínico Sándor Ferenczi* [*The Clinical Diary of Sándor Ferenczi*]. Buenos Aires: Conjetural.

Freud, S. (1893–1895). Estudios sobre la histeria. In Estudios sobre la Histeria (Breuer, J. y Freud, S.) (pp. 342–342).

Freud, S. (1897). "Draft M." In Ed. J. Strachey, *The Standard Edition of the Complete Psychological Works of Sigmund Freud*, Volume I. London: Hogarth Press.

Freud, S. (1909a). Family romances. In Ed. J. Strachey, *The Standard Edition of the Complete Psychological Works of Sigmund Freud*, Volume XIV. London: Hogarth Press.

Freud, S. (1909b). Notes upon a case of obsessional neurosis. In Ed. J. Strachey, *The Standard Edition of the Complete Psychological Works of Sigmund Freud*, Volume XIV. London: Hogarth Press.

Freud, S. (1911). Psycho-analytic notes on an autobiographical account of a case of paranoia (dementia paranoides). In Ed. J. Strachey, *The Standard Edition of the Complete Psychological Works of Sigmund Freud*, Volume XIV. London: Hogarth Press.

Freud, S. (1913). Psycho-analytic notes upon an autobiographical account of a case of paranoia (dementia paranoides). In Ed. J. Strachey, *The Standard Edition of the Complete Psychological Works of Sigmund Freud*, Volume XII. London: Hogarth Press.

Freud, S. (1914). On narcissism: An introduction. In Ed. J. Strachey, *The Standard Edition of the Complete Psychological Works of Sigmund Freud*, Volume XIV. London: Hogarth Press.

Freud, S. (1916). On transience. In Ed. J. Strachey, *The Standard Edition of the Complete Psychological Works of Sigmund Freud*, Volume XIV. London: Hogarth Press.

Freud, S. (1916–1917). The development of the libido and the sexual organizations, Lecture XXI. In Ed. J. Strachey, *The Standard Edition of the Complete Psychological Works of Sigmund Freud*, Volume XVI. London: Hogarth Press.

Freud, S. (1917). On transformations of instinct as exemplified in anal erotism. In Ed. J. Strachey, *The Standard Edition of the Complete Psychological Works of Sigmund Freud*, Volume XVII. London: Hogarth Press.

Freud, S. (1919). The 'Uncanny'. In Freud, S. (1919). *Introduction to Psycho-Analysis and the War Neuroses*. In Smith, I. (2000, 2007, 2010) *Freud – Complete Works*.

Freud, S. (1923a). The ego and the id. In Ed. J. Strachey, *The Standard Edition of the Complete Psychological Works of Sigmund Freud*, Volume XIX. London: Hogarth Press.

Freud, S. (1923b). The infantile genital organization. In Ed. J. Strachey, *The Standard Edition of the Complete Psychological Works of Sigmund Freud*, Volume XIX. London: Hogarth Press.

Freud, S. (1924). The dissolution of the Oedipus complex. In Ed. J. Strachey, *The Standard Edition of the Complete Psychological Works of Sigmund Freud*, Volume XIX. London: Hogarth Press.

Freud, S. (1925). Some psychical consequences of the anatomical distinction between the sexes. In Ed. J. Strachey, *The Standard Edition of the Complete Psychological Works of Sigmund Freud*, Volume XIX. London: Hogarth Press.

Freud, S. (1926). The Question of lay analysis. In Ed. J. Strachey, *The Standard Edition of the Complete Psychological Works of Sigmund Freud*, Volume XX. London: Hogarth Press.

Freud, S. (1931). Female sexuality. In Ed. J. Strachey, *The Standard Edition of the Complete Psychological Works of Sigmund Freud*, Volume XX. London: Hogarth Press.

Freud, S. (1933). Femininity, Lecture XXXIII. In Freud, S. (1933). *New Introductory Lectures on Psychoanalysis*. In Ed. J. Strachey, *The Standard Edition of the Complete Psychological Works of Sigmund Freud*, Volume XXI. London: Hogarth Press.

Freud, S. (1937). Analysis terminable and interminable. In Ed. J. Strachey, *The Standard Edition of the Complete Psychological Works of Sigmund Freud*, Volume XXIII. London: Hogarth Press.

Freud, S. (1941 [1921]). Psycho-analysis and telepathy. In Ed. J. Strachey, *The Standard Edition of the Complete Psychological Works of Sigmund Freud*, Volume XXIII. London: Hogarth Press.

Frydman, R. (1986). *L'irrésistible désir de naissance* [*The Irresistible Desire for Birth*]. Paris: Presses Universitaires de France.

Gilmore, D. D. (1999). *Hacerse hombre. Concepciones culturales de la masculinidad* [*Becoming a Man: Cultural Conceptions of Masculinity*]. Buenos Aires: Paidos.

Glocer Fiorini, L. (2001). *Lo femenino y el pensamiento complejo* [*The Feminine and the Complex Thinking*]. Buenos Aires: Lugar Editorial.

Green, A. (1992). *El complejo de castración* [*The Castration Complex*]. Buenos Aires: Paidós.

Groddeck, G. (1923). *The Book of the It*. In This, B. (1991). *Le Père: acte de naissance* [*The Father: An Act of Birth*]. Paris: Seuil.

Guerin, G. (1986). *L'enfant inconcevable* [*The Inconceivable Child*]. Paris: Acropole.

Hassoun, J. (1998). ¿Por qué se dice la virilidad? [Why do we say 'virility'?]. *Actualidad Psicológica*, "Lo masculino," #253 - May.

Héritier, F. (1992). Del engendramiento a la filiación [From procreation to filiation]. *Revista de Psicoanálisis con Niños y Adolescentes*, 22–31.

Héritier, F. (1996). *Masculin/Féminin. La pensée de la différence* [*Féminin/Masculine. The Thought of Difference*]. Paris: Editions Odile Jacob.

Hoad, T. F. (2003). *The Concise Oxford Dictionary of English Etymology*. Oxford: Oxford University.

Horney, K. (1922). On the genesis of the castration complex in women. *International Review of Psycho-Analysis*, 5, 50–65.

Jones, E. (1935). Early female sexuality. *The International Journal of Psycho-analysis*, 16, 263.

Klein, M. (1980). *Obras Completas [Complete Works]*. Buenos Aires: Paidos.

Lacan, J. (1957–1958). Las formaciones del inconsciente, seminario [Formations of the unconscious, seminar]. In S. Tubert (1991). *Mujeres sin sombra. Maternidad y tecnología [Women without a Shadow. Maternity and Technology]*. Madrid: Siglo XXI.

Lacan, J. (1966). La dirección de la cura y los principios de su poder [The direction of the treatment and the principles of its powers]. In S. Tubert (1991). *Mujeres sin sombra. Maternidad y tecnología [Women without a Shadow: Maternity and Technology]*. Madrid: Siglo XXI.

Langer, M. (1951). Maternidad y Sexo [*Maternity and Sexuality*]. Buenos Aires: Paidos.

Langer, M. (1982). "Oh, madre! Libérame de eso que llaman instinto maternal". [Oh, mother! Free me from that thing they call 'maternal instinct'"]. Buenos Aires: *Página12*, https://www.pagina12.com.ar/diario/psicologia/9-13777-2002-12-5.html

Laqueur T. W. (1992). *The Facts of Fatherhood*. In Eds B. Thorne and M. Yalom, *Rethinking the Family: Some Feminist Questions* (pp. 155–175). Boston: Northeastern University Press.

Le Breton, D. (1995). *Antropología del Cuerpo y Modernidad [Anthropology of the Body and Modernity]*. Buenos Aires: Nueva visión.

Morin, E. (1995). El pensamiento complejo. *Gedisa. Madrid.*

Nasio, J. D. (1991). La femineidad del padre [The father's femininity]. In M. Alizade, *Voces de Femineidad [Voices of Femininity]*. Buenos Aires: Alizade Ed.

Nerson-Sachs, C. (1995). De l'enfant imaginaire à l'enfant réel [From the imaginary child to the real child]. *Gynécologie et Obstetrique Psychosomatique*, #13, 27–33.

Perco, M. (2008). Personal communication.

Sahovaler, J. (1994). *Clase sobre Sexualidad Femenina [Lecture on Female Sexuality]*. given at the Gynecology Department of the Rivadavia Hospital, Buenos Aires.

Tajer, D. (2013). Diversidad y clínica psicoanalítica: apuntes para un debate [Diversity and psychoanalytic clinic: Notes for a debate]. In Ed. Fernández, A. & Siquera, W., *La diferencia desquiciada. Géneros y Diversidades Sexuales* (123–142). Buenos Aires: Editorial Biblos.

Török, M. (1964). El significado de la "envidia del pene" en la mujer. Translated by Paulette Michon Ferrand. *Revista Uruguaya de Psicoanálisis*, 6(4), 453–499.

Tort, M. (1992). El deseo frío. Procreación artificial y crisis de referencias simbólicas [Cold Desire. Artificial Procreation and the Crisis of Symbolic Reference Points]. Buenos Aires: Nueva Visión.

Tubert, S. (1991). *Mujeres sin sombra. Maternidad y tecnología [Women without a Shadow: Maternity and Technology]*. Madrid: Siglo XXI.

Vegetti Finzi, S. (1990). Désir de savoir et obscurité de l'origine [Desire to know and darkness of the origin]. In Ed. J. Testart, *Le magasin des enfants [The Children's Store]* (pp. 415–420). Paris: Gallimard.

Chapter 2

When Desire for a Child becomes Passion for a Child

On the frontiers of motherhood

In this chapter, we develop some ideas that have been taking shape over the years from listening to patients' consultations regarding infertility and medical-technological journeys. It is a clinical practice with unique characteristics, a practice that has led me to reflect on the desire for a child and its vicissitudes. This desire may place itself at the service of Eros or Thanatos.

We propose to analyse the following hypothesis: for women with reproductive disorders, desire for a child may become passion for a child. This passion may propel them to life, but may also traumatically become melancholy: the child, as a lost object or an object not found in real life, constitutes a unique, irreplaceable object that is a recipient of maternal love. This search for a child has specific characteristics: unusual intensity and fixation, even to the point of self-destruction (Alkolombre, 2008).

We have already discussed the notion of desire for a child in women and the way emotional constellations are presented in cases of female infertility. Passion for a child, as we develop it, manifests itself in clinical practice as an issue usually observed in women.

Passion is a descriptive rather than a metapsychological term; it has been made equivalent to falling in love: a loving passion. We may recall what Freud (1914) wrote about falling in love, which "(…) consists in a flowing-over of ego-libido onto the object," an imbalance in the economy of object libido that has "the power to remove repressions and reinstate perversions" (p. 100, Vol. XIV). *Passion* is a term Freud uses a few times. One of these is in the article "Leonardo Da Vinci and a Memory of His Childhood" (Freud, 1910), in which he describes passion as a driving force.

Passion is defined by emotional intensity and strong dependence on an object; it means to bear or endure love. It also denotes something passive, as opposed to movement and the exercise of will. According to Green (1980), it is about lovers who make you suffer to the point that you defend yourself from them through an alienating sacrifice. It is a powerful, incessant emotion that controls reason and guides behaviour.

DOI: 10.4324/9781003296713-4

The affective and representational overflow occurs in the context of phantasy and action. To experience passion is to be passive in relation to the object of passion, to expect everything from it: the restitution of narcissistic fulfilment and the joint satisfaction of Eros and Thanatos (Anzieu, 1980).

Green (1980) considers passion a basically affective phenomenon: love-passion/love-suffering. He observes that madness and passion are tied together throughout history as loving passions. In addition to *erotic passions*, he describes *narcissistic passions*, which have alienating effects on the individual who suffers from them.[1]

In madness, typically characterised as a disturbance of reason, Green continues, there is an affective component to be highlighted, a passionate component, which changes the relationship between the individual and the reality. It reminds us of the violence in little Hans' affects, his love for his mother and jealousy towards his father; these affects drive him "mad" with love; he is crazy in love. At this point, attending more to representations than to affects is an incomplete analysis, since it fails to recognise the suffering caused by an impossible love. Childhood love, as described by Freud in the initial epigraph, is boundless and demands exclusiveness. It is not satisfied with less than everything: such is the territory of loving passion.

Love and sexuality are part of life drives: Eros, as Freud (1920) explains in his final theory of drives: *life drives* and *death drives*. Green (1980) stresses that love necessarily entails a dimension of madness in the heart: love has a potential for passion.

What is the place of the *object of passion* and what is the relationship with that object? It is an exclusive, unique object that excludes all others from the field of cathexis. Paul Racamier (1980) states that the impassioned individual denies the object's autonomy and the autonomy of the real; the suffering that plagues impassioned individuals is that the object lives independently, thereby depriving them of the embodiments demanded by narcissistic needs. Therefore, the object of love in passion has the value of a narcissistic reference, untouchable and unchangeable.

The dead object—Racamier notes—is the most immutable of all objects of passion, since it is unalterable but can perfectly be manipulated. From a Judeo-Christian perspective, religious passion is oriented towards an ordeal, a passion related to love and suffering at the same time: loving and suffering through proofs of suffering sent by God. Parsons (2006) stresses the enormous cultural variety of religions, the rootedness of their traditions, and how different they are from each other. Some authors point out the spiritual function of psychoanalysis, showing in particular that self-knowledge, a goal of psychoanalysis, is intimately linked with the emotions of virtue (Symington, 2018). Following Freud, we learn that the origin of primitive religion is to be found in man's helplessness in relation to forces of impersonal nature. In turn, Perelberg (2015), following Freud's work, remarks on the link between the infant's experience of helplessness and traumata with excessive excitation.

Concerning the place of the object in passion, it may be partial or whole. An impassioned individual clings to it more or less exclusively and, most importantly, reorganises their perception of the world based on it (Green, 1980). It is a unique, excluding object, a hyper-cathected representation that alienates the ego: passion is blind. A unique, irreplaceable object—these are words used by Freud when describing the *infant's* relationship with its mother, as he describes it:

> The child's mother, who not only nourishes it but also looks after it and thus arouses in it a number of other physical sensations, pleasurable and unpleasurable. By her care of the child's body, she becomes its first seducer. In these two relations lies the root of a mother's importance, unique, without parallel, established unalterably for a whole lifetime as the first and strongest love object and as the prototype of all later love relations - for both sexes.
>
> (1940 [1938], p. 188)

In this paragraph, Freud stresses the relation with the first love object, the child's mother, who cathects, eroticises, nourishes, and provides pleasurable and unpleasurable sensations. These conditions make her a unique, irreplaceable object from which archetypes emerge throughout life. Despite real experience, this bond always gives the individual a feeling of being insufficient. It is the engine of psychic life and paves the way for mobilisation of the drive.

The experience of motherhood leads women to develop a specific constellation that Green (1980) calls *normal maternal madness.* Archaic anxieties are only the effect of narcissistic passions in which subject and object cannot be differentiated. This is the connection with the madness of love, a delusional aspect of transferences, erotic madness, and loving passions.

Green (1980) wonders: what is the force of drives, or the nature of fixation, in the end? They are no different from the intensity of the passion and the link to its object. And if we move on to child sexuality, he continues, the objects of passion must be found in partial objects taken from the mother's or the subject's body or in whole objects: parental imagos. For little Hans, a horse turns his anxieties into projections of his most intense emotions, his movements, and his strength: the drive, the passion.

How are these ideas connected to the passion for a child in a woman shifting from the desire for a child to the experience of what we propose to think of as a passion for a child?

A. Green (personal communication, October 2005) highlights that normal motherhood poses extraordinarily complex issues. During pregnancy, women usually develop a strong feeling of being everything for their child while the child becomes their only object, their only source of pleasure, care, and love. Women feel that they are giving and being everything to their babies at these early stages of motherhood. This bond loosens eventually but is always underlying the mother-child relationship (Green, 1980). These earliest times of motherhood constitute a central topic when we are discussing passion for a child.

M. Klein (1932) had a long-standing influence, introducing the infant's point of view into the early relationship. Later, Winnicott (1956) theorises from the mother's point of view. He argues that a baby cannot exist without its mother; at the same time, no mother can meet all the baby's needs in their early stages if the father does not play a supportive role. Winnicott develops the maternal emotional constellation through various concepts, one of which is *the good enough mother* (Winnicott, 1956).

In this regard, Kristeva (2011) points out that Freud's and Lacan's perspectives were mainly concerned with the paternal function but not the maternal function. She highlights that the maternal function is not a function but a passion. She argues that Winnicott's expression of *the good enough mother* does not address the violence of passion in maternal experience. Kristeva deepens the understanding of maternal passion by distinguishing passion from emotion. Motherhood is a passion in which emotions of attachment and aggression towards the child are transformed into love, dedication, and idealisation, together with a decrease in feelings of hate. Maternal passion develops in two phases: it begins with narcissistic withdrawal, and then it bonds with the object through projective identification sublimated as tenderness. This first stage of passion is internalised in relation to the object-child. The second stage is the mother's passion for her child, which takes place on the condition that the child ceases to be her double and is recognised as a subject and that the mother detaches herself from it so that the child acquires autonomy. She stresses that this movement of detachment is essential. She affirms that maternal passion is inhabited by the negative, which means that the inhibition of the drive allows the mother to transform these emotions into tenderness and care in the end. She concludes that maternal passion is the prototype of a love relationship.

Following Kristeva's ideas, women with passion for a child remain in the first internal stage of narcissistic withdrawal. The bifaceted part Kristeva describes is at the service not of tenderness and sublimation but rather at the service of passion. Detachment from the imaginary child, the second stage of the process, is absent. In this respect, the desire for a child in these passionate bonds remains fixed with great affective intensity. One of the characteristics of passion described by Cournut (1999) is the impossibility to work through mourning, which is why the child becomes an object that can be neither replaced nor sublimated. Women live with the promise that the following month, the following treatment, or the following doctor's appointment will be successful.

This persistent, insistent search for pregnancy is rooted, as discussed before, in the mother-child relationship as a prototype of the love relationship described by Freud: a unique, irreplaceable object Freud (1940): The search for pregnancy in the passion for a child is marked by attachment to the child to be born: an imaginary child conceived as a unique love object and recipient of maternal love. In these cases, the paternal function is often weak or absent.

Aulagnier (1979) highlights that passion belongs to a narcissistic and identification economy. Passion reveals the conflict between the ego and its ideals, as noted before. In the passion for a child, the maternal ideal is rooted not only in the woman's oedipal and narcissistic conflict but also in the place of motherhood in a patriarchal culture (Alkolombre, 2021). This woman's love for a child is fixed and depends on the absent object, as in the narcissistic passion where the idea "you will be mine or nobody's" prevails. In these cases, there is a narcissistic wound inflicted by gender and domestic violence.

The main features of the passion for a child are the intensity of emotions, persistence, and fixedness in the search for a child. Since there is no possibility of mourning (Cournut, 1999), patients undergo different reproductive treatments. In reference to this, Mali Mann (2018), in her book *Psychoanalytic Aspects of Assisted Reproductive Technology*, presents clinical cases of repeated IVF (in vitro fertilisation) trials. She analyses them in terms of their relation to repetition compulsion. She discusses how the acceptance of failure to conceive becomes in these cases a long process: an unfinished mourning in their lives. The use of multiple trials, Mann notes, is the central topic of discussion regarding narcissistic wounds. She stresses that unconscious trauma is the result of repetition compulsion of previously repressed trauma.

It is interesting to note Mann's emphasis on repetition compulsion in the face of the trauma of infertility. It is associated with previous traumas connected with the pre-oedipal bond with the mother. I believe that in the passion for a child, we are analysing the incessant and repetitive search for pregnancy through reproductive techniques in a compulsive manner. The most impressive case I dealt with was a couple who had undergone 17 unsuccessful in vitro fertilisations. Consequently, the understanding of the passionate relationship with the unborn child is that it is a narcissistic passion.

Along with these ideas, I argue that if we consider a woman's desire for a child to be at the theoretical core of femininity, we might consider motherhood essential to femininity. In that case, we risk basing our approach on a single, phallic woman's desire: the desire for a child. This passionate search for pregnancy might be critically understood through the naturalisation of the maternal ideal, in turn re-edited in Freudian theory. It is a conception of motherhood that relies on its idealisation and sacralisation, a maternal ideal prevalent in Freud's culture.

We know, moreover, that every historical period can raise questions that may be pondered. In regard to these ideas, Raphael-Leff (2015) notes that maternal ambivalence cannot be freely admitted in societies in which the idealisation of motherhood predominates. Various mechanisms operate to deal with prohibited feelings, increasing a main caregiver's tendency to polarise some hostile or rejected aspects of themselves or the environment by distorting, denying, splitting, and/or projecting. The title of her book, *The Dark Side of the Womb: Pregnancy, Parenting, and Persecutory Anxieties*, evokes a hidden aspect of motherhood, alluding to the Freudian idea of the woman as a dark continent. In her discussion, she deals with the experiences, fantasies, and fears that arise in different circumstances in the intrapsychic relationship between mother and foetus. Following Raphael-Leff's ideas, the passion for a child can be thought of as another dark side of motherhood when the desire for the imaginary and desired child is transformed in the mother's mind into a passion for a child.

When thinking about passion for a child within the dimension of narcissism, we observe ongoing tension between the ego and the ideals. The power of the ideals constitutes our subjectivity. Burin (1996) emphasises in work on gender theories the traits patriarchal culture leaves and its marks on the constitution of subjectivities. In turn, Dio Bleichmar (2002) remarks that if we want to study power in psychoanalytic terms, we cannot leave aside self-valorisation and the forms of social legality that sustain it.

Ideals are part of the narcissistic core in which the ego-ideal and the ideal ego coexist. Ideals are the link between the individual and the culture, which change according to the historical context. Ideals also determine what is expected of women and men in each time and place. Nowadays, in addition to traditional ideals of the heterosexual family, the universe of sexual diversity is included along with gender identities in families. In this respect, we are living in a time in which different models of families and gender identities coexist.

The motherhood paradigm is currently challenged, as we discussed earlier, by women's diverse experiences, present in our consulting rooms (Alkolombre, 2021). This introduces us to a new plural feminine desire that distances us from the idea of a sole desire for women. We see this movement in the diversity of desires that develop in new family configurations, some of them formed by reproductive techniques. These ideas lead us to rethink the maternal-feminine notion within a broader spectrum in the light of gender theories. As Tajer (2013) argues, the Freudian constitution of the desire for a child is revisited by gender theories. Therefore, this desire is thought of as an imaginary effect of the relation between motherhood and femininity historically constructed in modernity. I consider Tajer's ideas enable us to think of an extension of motherhood beyond the traditional Freudian view.

Glocer Fiorini (2001), in turn, discusses an alternative to the substitutive conception of the desire for the child: she extends the limits of the symbolic equation. She points out that although motherhood has natural support, it transcends it by inscribing itself in the register of culture within a symbolic universe. She also notes that psychoanalytic theory places motherhood within a phallic logic in which the child emerges as a symbolic substitute for a fundamental lack. The desire for a child in the woman is posited as a desiring-production, a conception of the child formulated beyond the lack posited within Freudian binarism.

When considering the passion for a child, we find several authors who put forward the idea of a child at all costs. Delaisi de Parseval and Janaud (1983) in their book *"L'enfant à tout prix"* present an essay on the medicalisation of the commodity of filiation. They highlight that they do not propose a critical view, but rather reflections on the use of reproductive techniques. In this regard, they emphasise that our society is living in a period in which there are deep changes concerning family representation systems, based on assisted reproduction. They note that during the 20th century, in particular since oral contraception, the place of the child has acquired a new meaning: it represents an affective and narcissistic capital, which has consequences for both children and parents. They point out that couples use contraceptive pills until they decide to become parents, months or years later. In these cases, they are living in a sort of omnipotence with the illusion of control over their reproductive capacities. However, as time goes on and pregnancy does not arrive, they feel the anxiety that often accompanies the desire to have a child. Thus, they wonder about the "child at all costs," that is, those born as a result of a "great struggle" against infertility. These authors note that the idea of control occupies a central place in the patients' reflections, since it is no longer a child that couples make—or find difficult to make— but something that, in phantasy, more closely resembles faeces, as in Freud's equivalence faeces-penis-child-money-gift. And when pregnancy does not come, it is more constipation than infertility. Together with the idea that the child should be, from an emotional point of view, a loving project with narcissistic and anal components which, although present, should not be dominant. However, they affirm that in practice the perspective of control "at all costs" becomes dominant.

Another author who analyses the idea of the child at any cost is Ansermet (2018). In his book *The Art of Making Children* (2018), he notes that the child is related to the wish to make something immortal and to transcend. Regarding this topic, Abadi (1960) stresses that what is central in life is its inexorable race towards death, pointing out that the most biological of the defences that work against death anxiety is procreation: perpetuation through the child. He affirms that the child is a key piece between life and death, as a transmitter of a lineage and transcendence. Ansermet, in turn, argues that when a child is desired at all costs through reproductive techniques, in many cases the desire for a child is lost. In these cases, the desire for a child is blurred because it is under the imperative that it must be "at all costs." He affirms something that seems a tautology but makes sense: the desire to have a child at any cost can take the place of the desire to have a child.

Related to this topic, Tubert (2010) points out that the search for a child at all costs is supported by the desire for a child, which legitimises it. She notes, however, that women who undergo assisted fertility treatment build their desire into an obsession in their discourse on the techniques. She starts with the idea of identification with the cultural ideals of motherhood, associating the maternal with the feminine. Tubert also points out that during assisted fertility treatment women lose their position as desiring subjects in order to passively incorporate the medical discourse that reduces them to their reproductive organs.

However, I consider that thinking about a child at all costs is not enough to think about these cases our clinical practice is presenting. The hypothesis I postulate is that passion for a child is one of the destinies of the desire for a child and that it develops on the basis of the narcissistic-passion axis.

Destinies of motherhood: Passion for a child

The search for a child puts all the libidinal economy into play; it cherishes the dimensions of love and identity. For men, it means reaffirming their potency and virility, and for women, it means the confirmation of their femininity. All this applies to the more traditional version of masculine-feminine.

From the psychoanalytic perspective, among the three paths that Freud proposes for women, the one corresponding to femininity sends us to motherhood (Freud, 1933). As we analysed before, thinking of it as the only way out, as a hegemonic desire, may induce psychoanalytic listening to accompany these passionate searches for children, many of the technological ones, without guessing the hypo-cathected processes associated with the thanatic aspects these journeys usually entail.

Women who undergo assisted fertilisation treatments time and again, generally unsupported, arrive at their consultation emotionally devastated, feeling empty as well as desperate to continue. They are always promised that the next treatment will be successful, that the baby is coming.

When desire comes into play, some passion is always present, but the delicate balance between what can and cannot be achieved, as well as the prevailing randomness of biology, places women at a crossroads. Between the possibility and the impossibility of fulfilling this desire, as regards infertility and reproductive techniques, Aulagnier (1992) writes that renouncing the desire is equivalent to a psychic death but being unable to accept the limits on its fulfilment may have equally catastrophic results. A passion may propel us to life, but a passion may also become melancholy.

The passion for a child reveals the pain as well as the imaginary whirlwind swirling around ideas about the absent, missing object and the affects associated with it. Passion is also a part of love, and its power, its spirit, is fundamentally positive. The risk lies in being unable to discern the suffering, thanatic aspects of passion that usually appear fused in these medical-technological journeys, and to work with them. It is a passion that contains the driving force of life, but also the abyss of nothingness.

In the passion for a child, strength comes from the signs of their absence, found in the tension of the wait. For these patients, the long-awaited child, like a hidden sun, leaves the entire universe in shadows. As already noted, the search for a child may be driven by desire or passion. Therefore, passion for a child is located on the borders of motherhood, between a desire for motherhood and a "maternal neurosis" or maternal madness: the wished-for child becomes the woman's fancied guarantee of survival. This search has specific characteristics as I mentioned, and it has an unusual intensity and fixation, even to the point of self-destruction.

I now introduce the clinical case that led me to conceive the hypothesis of a transformation of desire for a child into a passion for a child.

Marcela was 28 years old at the time of the consultation. She had been married to Ricardo for a year, and she mentioned an unsatisfactory sex life.

She was the middle sister of three women. She was born a year later than her older sister, who was closer to her mother. Marcela had always had a distant relationship with her father, an extremely introverted, cold man. She remembered him sitting in the dark in the living room, in silence or watching TV for whole afternoons.

In her adolescence, her exogamous journey was closely monitored by her parents. Marcela did not confront them due to her submission and her great need for love and recognition.

For a long time, I listened to Marcela talk about her desire for a child, her sorrow. I worked hard with her to understand the root cause of her complaints, the reasons behind her powerful fixation on her search for pregnancy, her relation to femininity, and her history.

It was almost a ritual; for some time, we made progress in understanding the situation, and she seemed able to decentre and think of herself as someone fertile for life, but before long, we were retracing our steps. At times, I found myself thinking of how powerless I was to help her. Every month, it was always the same announcement with similar words:

> This month I haven't gotten pregnant ... I'll never make it. Why does this have to happen to me? Many women don't want to get pregnant. Maybe the obstacle makes the desire stronger in me. I don't know. I'd have one after the other. It's the only thing that could fulfil me, having babies. I'd like to have many.

She repeatedly expressed feeling guilty for not being a mother. These complaints evoked older complaints: getting less attention from her mother, being given little room because she was the middle sister, and having always felt left aside. As a matter of fact, her room was a passage, almost a hallway between the two other bedrooms.

I found myself thinking about the specific features of the child as a love object: it is unconditional, considering the basic asymmetry of mother-child bonding, and is also a part of the woman's body, the seat of maternal narcissism; a special love object. And in this case, it was someone who was only for her, not to be shared with other people; exclusively for her, exclusively for the baby.

Working with Marcela, I initially thought that hyper-cathexis of the reproductive function, the difficult relationship with her mother, and increasing female castration anxiety explained the intensity of the effects involved: her difficulties for thinking, the repeated crises she went through every month when faced with the impossibility of getting pregnant.

After a year of therapy, she started an assisted fertilisation treatment (in vitro fertilisation[2]). Before she started the therapy, she had tried many intra-uterine inseminations but did not manage to get pregnant. This time she got pregnant, but I noticed that her anxiety was not dispelled. She started to be afraid that her pregnancy would not go well and that something bad would happen. Again, it all revolved around the child to be born, not the pregnancy that will not come.

She went through the first stage of pregnancy with nausea and vomiting, which accounted for the ambivalence and anxiety she experienced in this new situation.

She also demanded increasingly more assistance from her mother: help with housework and keeping her company. She even asked her mother to wash her hair because finding hairs on her pillow after brushing made her nauseous, an issue more related to an almost delirious displacement. Some intensity of passion was present.

She started to behave like a baby who wanted to satisfy primary needs; she became a daughter-baby to be taken care of, who called for her mother. Her mother even accompanied her as far as my consulting room many times and then went to pick her up.

In the end, she had an uneventful pregnancy from an organic point of view. However, in terms of emotions, she had to face and work through periods of much anguish and anxiety that continued once her daughter was born.

This led me to think that this search for fusion with the imaginary child reproduced part of her fusional bond with her mother which failed in Marcela's childhood. It was unfinished business.

Thus, we observe a two-phase process: a pre-oedipal phase linked to her relationship with her body and her mother's body, and the oedipal phase in its negative variant, where she battles against her sisters for her mother's attention. The father figure is more blurred, neither cutting the bond with her mother nor reassuring her of her femininity. He is an absent father for Marcela.

Clinical practice enabled me to reflect on cases similar to Marcela's perseverance in diverse, sometimes bloody procedures, years spent, depression, and also two distinct features: fixation, a persistent search, and affective intensity. Can all these features be explained only by the maternal ideal, female castration anxiety, and pre-oedipal conflict?

Is it the *child at all cost* as Delaisi de Parseval and Janaud (1983), Tubert (1991), and Ansermet (2018) posit?

However, in my clinical experience, I did consider it from a narcissistic-impassioned perspective. I pursued another avenue that considers libidinal withdrawal and efforts to re-create a state of fusion with the original object via motherhood: the child to be born. Also, *His Majesty the Baby* (Freud, 1914) or *Their Majesty the Baby*[3,4] are associated not only with transcendence and legacy but also rooted in the maternal ideal—as the only and unique destiny for women: being a mother.

Freud argues that a lover's feelings are extinguished by bodily ailments. But he adds that "in the last resort, we must begin to love in order not to fall ill" (1914, p. 85). This imperative comes together with the mandate of the maternal ideal in femininity that reinforces this destiny.

By this path I arrived at the hypothesis: *for these women, desire for a child turns into passion for a child, the latter constituting a unique object, the recipient of that love. Passion is the shape the suffering ego takes when subjected to the ideal of motherhood* (Alkolombre, 2020).

Passion arises in the relationship with that "absent" child in a fixed, unceasing, excessive, and demanding way. Like the childhood love that Freud described: boundless, exclusive, not content with less than all.

Infertility is experienced as a narcissistic wound as Marcela says: "Why does this have to happen to me?"

In passion for a child, the expectation of a "pregnancy-baby" is heavily cathected, establishing an inner dialogue with that absence and permanently questioning the body. There is a demand, an urgency to change reality, trying to overcome the barrier they have encountered.

Reflecting on it and moving away from the concrete situation become difficult tasks. Infertility appears as something "unconceivable-unthinkable."

As regards the object of passion, Aulagnier (1992) stresses that the object of passion is an irreplaceable, necessary object because it is the answer to a desire that has become a necessity. The term passion excludes the shared or mutual passionate relationship (1979).

The passion for a child translates into "living for" getting pregnant. Pregnancy is assigned a place of privilege, idealised, and free of conflict. Pregnancy also represents putting an end to the frustration of infertility.

Motherhood remains as an ideal, as something exclusive, which gives pleasure and, as an absence, causes extreme suffering. The present is undervalued; all that matters is the future, the wait, and the expectation of pleasure. The present is grief without death. Passion turns towards the absent child and, at this point, we confuse it with the idea of a lost object, an object that is absent because it is not yet a part of reality.

When the woman aims to give it an existence, the child does not appear. It is a kind of hallucinatory desire to bring the child into existence (A. Green, personal communication, October 2005). A priceless child, since there is an attempt to screen an image of what the woman would like to have: herself and her baby.

Passion for a child is an affective movement that derives from the desire to give life to that child, as Green added when I supervised with him. In this way, the endless search itself serves as reassurance for a weakened narcissism.

When a patient says that it is "the only thing that fulfils me," meaning the child to be born, she is talking about something that is not replaceable, about something necessary for her, because it responds to a desire that has become a need. Passion joins helplessness. She might also say: "Without the pregnancy, I am nothing," while hiding her defencelessness.

The pregnancy is going to redeem her and make up for everything she has suffered. The other one, the child of her dreams, is the one who restores wounded narcissism. It allows her to run away from her powerlessness, from her impossibility.

Fusion with this maternal ideal, representing the ideal, narcissistic ego that comes from primary identifications, allows for the search for narcissistic satisfaction in the face of dissatisfaction due to the inability to find the object.

In clinical practice, transference is saturated by the primacy of affect, of suffering for an object presented as impossible and unattainable.

The impassioned individual's place has some contradictory aspects: we may see them as if they were a star in a certain situation, but in others they seem to be a victim going through intense suffering: the passive aspect of pursuing an ideal.

Passion regularly includes a denial of judgement that would tend to diminish the prestige and value of the object of passion, previously cathected as an ideal. When Freud describes falling in love, he notes the phenomenon of idealisation of the object, which is eventually treated as the ego. It is a passionate love because "what possesses the excellence which the ego lacks for making it an ideal, is loved" (Freud, 1914, p. 101).

The object replaces the ego ideal and, in that state, the individual increasingly renounces their own complaints to the point of self-sacrifice. They surrender to the object that has become magnificent. Freud (1921) also compares this state to hypnosis, since in both cases there is a relationship between someone more powerful and another person in a state of dependence and abandonment. Aulagnier (1979) defines passion as an asymmetrical relationship.

What is important about passion for a child is that, due to fixation, it does not stop, but persists and insists, even beyond the principle of pleasure. It also contains, as said at the beginning of this chapter, some of the childhood love that is always intense and boundless, passionate.

The child as a passion unveils an excess and, as with every passion, it marks our lives significantly. It is an excess of expectation of pleasure as well as an excess of the possibility of suffering.

Understanding passion: The narcissistic axis

The child for parents is a representant of narcissism: His *Majesty the Baby*. As we said before, the immortality of the ego takes refuge in the child, the most sensitive point of the narcissistic system. The child who has not yet arrived is the one who does not reinforce parental narcissism: they are child-less parents..

By going through a passionate relationship, the *infant* finds love. It is an initiatory bond which is fusional and essential for the constitution of the subject. Aulagnier (1979) mentions that for this reason we always feel nostalgia for the excess of pleasure experienced in the encounter with the first object of passion. At the same time, we feel anxiety in relation to re-experiencing such a relationship and again feeling the excess of suffering when we had to overcome it.

As mentioned earlier, the child's ego passionately cathects the mother's ego: it confirms that the mother is doubly unique and irreplaceable (Freud, 1937). She is the first and most intense love object, the archetype of subsequent bonds. In the passionate bond, the choice of a primary drive object is revalidated. Therefore, passion for a child possesses a double inscription: from the initiatory bond with their mother and from the bond to be formed with a child, with one's offspring.

The child's place is in the field of narcissism from the perspective of psychoanalysis, which ensures the parents' immortality and allows them to project the parents' desires. As Freud puts it: "Parental love, which is so moving and at the bottom so childish, is nothing but the parents' narcissism born again" (1914, p. 91).

A narcissistic bond can be sustained at any cost, which leads me to think about the power of narcissism and its counterpart, helplessness.

Passion reveals the narcissistic aspect. Freud (1914, p. 90) argues that each individual has two object-choice possibilities that correspond, at the same time, to two primary sexual objects: themselves (*narcissistic choice*) and their mother or the person who nurses, protects, and cares for them (*attachment* or *anaclitic choice*).

In a narcissistic choice, individuals love themselves and need not so much to love as to be loved. They love what they are, what they were, what they would like to be, or the person that was a part of themselves.

As mentioned in the chapter on the desire for a child, loving a child entails a passage of narcissistic libido to the object of love. As the object libido is not satisfied because pregnancy does not occur, the desired object is nothing but an absence. Nor is narcissistic satisfaction obtained from fulfilling the maternal ideal. There is instead a return to a narcissistic position.

Sacrificial movements begin so that the individual recovers a more satisfactory self-image. It incarnates the ideal, even without protection or limits when facing extreme situations.

In these cases, there is a demand to adapt to that maternal ideal. No type of symbolic substitution is admitted, and there is no grieving over limits encountered. Other ways to access motherhood are not valid. In this context, there is an aggressive component at work through the sacrificial body. The body must do what is expected of it.

In passion, desire escapes the drive and is fictitiously trapped in the object. Everything it does and asks for is fair and irreproachable because it has been placed as an ideal. Passion may become melancholy; the missing object may devour the ego. When object choice is not predominantly narcissistic, the rejection and disappointment it causes may lead to progressive detachment in the search for more satisfactory bonds and may enable mourning. However, narcissistic fragility increases the individual's vulnerability and facilitates the emergence of a passion.

Through passion, the ego's exceptional quality is put to the test as a source of pleasure. This is how "miraculous" pregnancies occur, attained thanks to all sorts of endless sacrifices. But reality is not always satisfactory; therefore, passion's ideal is usually frustrating when confronted with reality.

Alienation in a passion for a child may work as a narcissistic defence against the suffering inherent in mourning. In these cases, working through the grief caused by infertility would enable recovery of the desire for a child. Otherwise, the way out is sacrificial passion.

Another issue is the place of man in these "maternal passions." Many times, it is often men with an absent profile who do not interfere in the woman's relationship in the search for a pregnancy.

They are men whose wives displace their sexuality onto motherhood— they are mothers rather than women, and their husbands stay by their side accepting this place. They are wanted not so much for being men as for being fathers of the child to be born.

In Marcela's case, her husband left her alone with her *passion for a child*, which extended far beyond the birth: her child slept in her bedroom until she was one and a half, and the couple took a long time to resume their sex life.

The man's inclusion becomes fundamental and guarantees the mother's separation from the child. It enables the man to offer himself as an object of drive satisfaction so that the child is not left as the woman's only possible love object.

The father's absence also blocks confrontation with a thirdness and provides a diagnostic factor to explain a woman's tendency to search for a child in a passionate and fusional relationship. Hence the importance of including a link perspective in these consultations.

Attachment and sacrifice in passion

The positive aspect of passion is linked with the work of binding, an attempt to heal "a protective psychic bridge" (Alizade, 1999) the individual recreates to establish a new alliance with life, to better endure the absence of the missing love object.

The desire for a child becomes the guarantor of the survival of the maternal phantasm. Freud writes about a way to control these "quantities":

> Working them over in the mind helps remarkably towards an internal draining of excitations incapable of direct external discharge, or when such a discharge is momentarily undesirable. In the first instance, however, it is a matter of indifference whether this internal process of working-through is in relation to real or imaginary objects. The difference appears only later if the turning of the libido onto unreal objects (introversion) has led to its being dammed up.
>
> (Freud, 1914, p. 85)

The positive aspect of passion lies in relation with this processing, where excitations "incapable of direct external discharge" remain as a phantasy. It is this damming up, the hyper-cathexis, that fixates the object and makes it necessary. This makes us wonder if we can find a destiny of sublimation in maternal passion, the chance to work through grief, and re-cathect a different project, another path to motherhood.

We may observe that the more fixated the passion for a child, the smaller the chance of displacement and resolution, for example, through adoption.

The negativity of passion is connected to a sacrificial position in the passionate search for a child. It is the *dark side*, a thanatic side that impedes the establishment of bindings that may form the foundations for working through grief.

Because of their psychic cost, these motherhoods involve degradation and alienation. It is a way of suffering that demands joy in its fixation and intensity.

In passionate searches for children, a sacrificial attitude is installed. These patients risk everything for a child: their bodies, their mind, their health, and their money. In Marcela, we find that melancholy appears in reverse, as subjugation to the object that has become grandiose.

Aulagnier (1979) contends that the object of passion is cathected by two drives: Eros and Thanatos. Pleasure in the wait and the risk of death are both present.

The individual recognises the absence but preserves the certainty of finding it in the future. As mentioned above, Cournut (1999) argues that passion in a relationship is summed up in the presence or the absence of another person: in the pleasure of the presence and unpleasure of the absence.

The violence of surrender to the ideal is proportionate to the violence implied in the narcissistic wound. In Marcela, as in many unquestioned surrenders to reproductive techniques, the passionate search for a child remains a complex scenario in which the presence and absence of a missing object unfold.

The final result may also become hate towards the woman's own body, its mistreatment, or a masochistic search for mistreatment through many medical-technological procedures.

Beneath this unrestricted, conflict-free love, we may glimpse a suffocated ambivalence: intense hatred for this child who does not arrive and is a source of frustration. This hatred is expressed by intolerance towards pregnant women, childbirth: the presence of what the woman longs for.

Passion remains in a position opposite to reason. It shares excess with madness. It is associated with an attitude of commitment that takes emotion as far as possible. This attitude is often concealed in our culture by the extreme idealisation of "maternal love" (Badinter, 1980).

In conclusion, we may say that unlike desire, sustained by drives, passion depends on an object. The passion for a child depends on a narcissistically cathected object.

In clinical practice, passion appears as a persistent, insistent search for a child "beyond the principle of pleasure," added to the libidinal withdrawal and reactivation of the female castration complex produced by infertility.

Passion has two aspects: a positive aspect—attempted binding and attachment—and a negative, sacrificial aspect, the action of a death drive, related to sacrificial behaviours and some medical-technological journeys.

This hypo-cathexis leaves no traces since a certain social consensus usually makes the woman's behaviour invisible: a woman drops her activities one by one because she is "dedicated to getting pregnant." The risk is that this movement towards psychic isolation may produce a void in the group of objects that are part of her representational capital, leaving her at the mercy of the death drive.

Here, we are defining the boundaries between desire for a child and passion for a child. A difference that may be expressed this way: "having" a child or "being" by means of a child. Passion does not allow giving up on gratifying its desire because it implies a narcissistic wound and facing lacks.

The search for a child as a passion comes with a certain "naturalness" of a typically feminine desire. Although psychoanalytic listening provides various theoretical lines and points of view, a woman's field of desire seems to be almost completely saturated by motherhood. In this regard, we ask an open question for further reflection: how does the psychoanalyst's point of view affect the case, and what is the analyst's framework?

As a passion, the child is born in an atmosphere of love and may become a destiny in a woman's life.

In the fluctuating borders of desire for a child, motherhood reveals diverse paths of desire in women.

Notes

1 In his article *Passions et destins des passions*, Green (1980) draws a very important distinction between madness and psychosis. He states that there is madness, as a passionate affect, in every transference. Psychotic transference is different: its only goal is to destroy the analytical setting. Green defines madness as a disturbance of reason, stressing the affective-passionate component, which changes the individual's relationship with reality and alienates them. He also observes that transference is initially recognised as a loving transference—a false connection—and emphasises that this is where loving passion resurfaces.

2 In vitro fertilisation (IVF): consists of ovarian stimulation, ova extraction (via aspiration or puncture), and fertilisation in the laboratory by the natural action of capacitated sperm. Afterwards, if embryos form (one or more), they develop in appropriate environments until they are placed in the uterus (embryo transfer, ET) (Perco, personal communication, 2008).

3 Italics are mine.

4 This is an important topic, among other things, due to the success rate (approximately 25–30%) of reproductive techniques, which presents a difficult path forward. Moreover, the standard pregnancy rate for a healthy couple is around 30% for each cycle (Perco, personal communication, 2008).

References

Abadi, M. (1960). *Renacimiento de Edipo: la vida del hombre en la dialéctica del adentro y del afuera* [*Rebirth of Oedipus: Man's Life in the Dialect between Inside and Outside*]. Buenos Aires: Nova.

Alizade, M. (1999). *Feminine Sensuality*. London: Karnac.

Alkolombre, P. (2004). Psicoanálisis y relaciones de género en fertilidad asistida [Psychoanalysis and gender relations in assisted fertility]. In Eds M. Alizade and T. Lartigue, *Psicoanálisis y relaciones de Género* (pp. 79–93). Buenos Aires: Lumen.

Alkolombre, P. (2008). *Deseo de hijo. Pasión de hijo: esterilidad y técnicas reproductivas a la luz del psicoanálisis* [*Desire for a Child. Passion for a Child. Infertility and Reproductive Techniques in the Light of Psychoanalysis*]. Buenos Aires: Letra Viva.

Alkolombre, P. (2009). Nuevos escenarios masculinos en fertilidad asistida: un vientre para él [New male scenarios in assisted fertility: A womb for him]. In *Libro del VIII Diálogo COWAP IPA: El padre. Clínica, género, posmodernidad* (pp. 153–160). Lima: Peruvian Psychoanalytic Society.

Alkolombre, P. (2020). Pasión de hijo [Passion for a child]. In *Diccionario de Psicoanálisis Argentino* (pp. 355–358). Buenos Aires: Argentine Psychoanalytic Association.

Alkolombre, P. (2021). The maternal-feminine: Scenarios in transformation psycho-analysis and gender perspectives. In *Psychoanalytic Explorations of What Women Want Today* (pp. 161–171). Routledge.

Ansermet, F. (2018). *The Art of Making Children: The New World of Assisted Reproductive Technology.* London and New York: Routledge.

Anzieu, D. (1980). "Une passion pour rire: L' esprit" [A passion for laughing: The spirit]. In Collectif (1980), *La passion, Nouvelle Revue de Psychanalyse (#21)* [*The Passion, New Journal of Psychoanalysis*] (p. 165). Paris: Gallimard. *aternidad* [*Paternity*]. Buenos Aires: Kargieman, p. 32.

Aulagnier, P. (1979). *Los destinos del placer: alienación, amor, pasión* [*The Destiny of Pleasure: Alienation, Love, Passion*]. Buenos Aires: Paidós.

Aulagnier, P. (1992). 'Qué deseo, de qué hijo?' [What desire? For what child?]. *Revista de Psicoanálisis con Niños y Adolescentes*, (3), 45–49.

Badinter, E. (1980). *L'amour de plus* [*Love More*]. Paris: Flammarion..

Burin, M. (1996). *Género, psicoanálisis, subjetividad* [*Gender, Psychoanalysis, Subjectivity*] (pp. 61–99). Buenos Aires: Paidós.

Castoriadis-Aulagnier, P. (1977). *La violencia de la interpretación* [*The violence of inter-pretation*]. Buenos Aires: Amorrortu.

Cournut, J. (1999). L'énergie de la passion [The energy of passion]. In Ed. J. André, *De la passion* [*Passion*] (pp. 7–26). France: PUF.

Delaisi de Parseval, G., & Janaud, A. (1983). *L' enfant à tout prix: Essai sur la médical-isation du lien de filiation* [*Children at All Costs. Essay on the Medicalization of the Link of Parentage*]. Paris: Du Seuil.

Dio Bleichmar, E. (2002). Sexualidad y género: nuevas perspectivas en el psicoanálisis contemporáneo. *Aperturas psicoanalíticas, 11*.

Freud, S. (1910). Leonardo Da Vinci and a memory of his childhood. In Ed. J. Strachey, *The Standard Edition of the Complete Psychological Works of Sigmund Freud*, Volume XIII. London: Hogarth Press.

Freud, S. (1914). On narcissism: An introduction. In Ed. J. Strachey, *The Standard Edition of the Complete Psychological Works of Sigmund Freud*, Volume XIV. London: Hogarth Press.

Freud, S. (1920). Beyond the pleasure principle. In Ed. J. Strachey, *The Standard Edition of the Complete Psychological Works of Sigmund Freud*, Volume XVIII. London: Hogarth Press.

Freud, S. (1921). Group psychology and the analysis of the ego. In Ed. J. Strachey, *The Standard Edition of the Complete Psychological Works of Sigmund Freud*, Volume XVIII. London: Hogarth Press.

Freud, S. (1933). "Feminity," Lecture XXXIII. In Ed. J. Strachey, *The Standard Edition of the Complete Psychological Works of Sigmund Freud*, Volume XX. London: Hogarth Press.

Freud, S. (1937). Analysis terminable and interminable. In Ed. J. Strachey, *The Standard Edition of the Complete Psychological Works of Sigmund Freud*, Volume XXIII. London: Hogarth Press.

Freud, S. (1940). An outline of psycho-analysis. In Ed. J. Strachey, *The Standard Edition of the Complete Psychological Works of Sigmund Freud*, Volume XXIII. London: Hogarth Press.

Glocer Fiorini, L. (2001). *Lo femenino y el pensamiento complejo* [*The Feminine and the Complex Thinking*]. Buenos Aires: Lugar Editorial.

Green, A. (1980). Passions et destins des passions [Passions and destinies of passions]. *Nouvelle Revue de Psychanalyse*, *21*, 25.

Klein, M. (1932). *El Psicoanálisis de Niños*. Buenos Aires: Paidós.

Kristeva, Julia. (2011). "Motherhood today." *Revue française de psychosomatique*, *40*(2), 43–51. DOI: 10.3917/rfps.040.0043. URL: https://www.cairn-int.info/journal-revue-francaise-de-psychosomatique-2011-2-page-43.htm

Mann, M. (2018). *Psychoanalytic Aspects of Assisted Reproductive Technology*. Routledge.

Parsons, R. (2006). Ways of transformation. *Psychoanalysis and Religion in the 21st Century. Competitors or Collaborators* (pp. 117–131). New York.

Perelberg, R. J. (2015). On excess, trauma, and helplessness: Repetitions and transformations. *The International Journal of Psychoanalysis*, *96*(6), 1453–1476.

Racamier, P. C. (1980). "De l'objet-non-objet. Entre folie, psychose et pasión" ["Of the object-not-object. Between madness, psychosis and passion"]. *Nouvelle Revue de Psychanalyse*, 21, 235–241.

Raphael-Leff, J. (2015). *The Dark Side of the Womb: Pregnancy, Parenting, and Persecutory Anxieties*. London: Anna Freud Centre.

Symington, N. (2018). *Emotions and Spirit. Questioning the Claims on Psychoanalysis and Religion*. London: Routledge.

Tajer, D. (2013). Diversidad y clínica psicoanalítica: apuntes para un debate [Diversity and the psychoanalytic clinic: Notes for a debate]. In Ed. A. Fernández y W. Siquera, *La diferencia desquiciada. Géneros y Diversidades Sexuales* (pp. 123–142). Buenos Aires: Editorial Biblios.

Tubert, S. (1991). *Mujeres sin sombra. Maternidad y tecnología* [*Women without a Shadow: Maternal Desire and Assisted Reproductive Technologies*]. Madrid: Siglo XXI.

Tubert, S. (2010). Los ideales culturales de la feminidad y sus efectos sobre el cuerpo de las mujeres [Cultural ideals of femininity and their effects on women's bodies]. *Quadernos de psicología*, *12*(2), 161–174.

Winnicott, W. (1956). *Escritos de psiquiatría y psicoanálisis*. Barcelona, Buenos Aires, México: Paidós.

Part II

Techniques in the Light of Psychoanalysis

Chapter 3

Into Psychoanalytic Clinical Work

About the erogenous body in infertility

In this chapter, we deal with a key topic for our clinical work in the field of infertility: the place of the erogenous body and the biological body. These scenarios are part of the search for a child.

"I want to have a child because I'm afraid I can't have a child," Marina said as she agitatedly arrived at my office for her first interview. She did not notice the insistence in her words. She was only 27 years old and had been married for three years. She was now facing the question of why she had not yet been able to get pregnant. She was distressed.

Consultations similar to Marina's are common and reflect clinical work in which conscious and unconscious aspects emerge in the search for a pregnancy. It all starts as if the lips of some patients said "yes," but their bodies said "no." Many times, analysts are asked to find a cure for paradoxes in the complex mind-body bond that interact with fantasies and narratives expressed in clinical work.

We may remember that psychoanalysis begins with the body. This is how the symptoms of hysterical conversion led Freud when studying cases of hysteria to discover the erogenous body, which does not match the anatomy of the body as described by medicine (Freud, 1983–1985). This reveals representations incompatible with the ego which lead to functional disorders. In his work, Freud introduced the concept of *drive*, which is bodily in essence. It arises from anaclisis in the erogenous zones, and its object is the child's own body or that of others. Therefore, the drive functions as the psychical representative of the somatic. It is also defined as the amount of energy demanded from psychic processes as a consequence of its binding with the body. In turn, Green (1980) argues that the energy demanded from psychic processes comes from the body to which it is bound; in other words, psychic processes are materialised in the body.

The body plays a central role due to its double condition as a subject and also an object of the external world. It is the body that feels pleasure and pain, and it is the body that falls ill. Freud (1914) explains in his article

DOI: 10.4324/9781003296713-6

On Narcissism: An Introduction, that libido and the ego's interest converge in organic illness and become indistinguishable.

Piera Aulagnier (1994) holds that more than one identity is established between our mental representation of our body and our real body and that each subject passes judgement on their own. She adds that the body may be loved or hated and that it asks to be repaired and taken care of by another person.

From Freud's (1930) standpoint, the most interesting ways to find protection against suffering involve trying to have influence over one's own body. This is linked to the different ways in which we experience suffering when faced with the difficulty of conceiving, which is in some cases seen as an adverse fate or as punishment associated with conscious or unconscious guilt. When this fear and guilt is analysed at an individual level, it becomes a powerful trigger of personal situations that unfold during the analysis.

The woman's body

> I try not to think about it ... I don't know ... My mom had five children. To make things worse, my friends get pregnant out of thin air. Because, you know. If I want something, I buy it, or if I see something I like, I try to get it. This I don't know! I cannot understand it ... I have terrible cramps during my period.

In my first sessions with Marta, I felt as if she were trying to say and also not to say something about herself. Her cramps were the only possible record of her experience of pain; a pain that was expressed and assigned meaning through the body. However, another pain was not present: the psychic suffering with which she lived. Her words reflected her lack of understanding and perplexity about why she could not yet get pregnant.

How can we address the problem of the body in all its density and fleshiness? In this case, the problem is a body that does not respond to expectations. The fact that the body does not do what it should do is seen as unfathomable, a narcissistic wound. Questions such as "Why me? I don't know why!" are frequent in these analyses.

A common denominator in these cases is how the body's *not-doing* impacts and surprises patients. This *not-doing* renders the body an enigma and alters the body-subject relation. A particular tension is thereby created between the body and the desire for a child, whose cathexis only grows as time goes by.

The imaginary of a *predictable body* that may be modified by medical-technological interventions is faced with an unpredictable body tied to the laws of biology and also to expressions of the unconscious (Alkolombre, 2008).

The anatomical body is studied, undergoing different medical treatments that are uniquely and singularly thought and imaginarised by each woman.

Infertility appears unexpectedly, even if the idea of not having children existed as a fantasy. However, when reality confirms difficulties in conceiving, the impact is different. Every woman frequently faces more primitive anxieties, the body becomes an enigma, and a new subject-body relation begins to develop. This is clearly seen in this short clinical vignette: Graciela said, "I feel I've been living in a bubble ... and now I'm faced with all this ... We used to think we needed to use protection [birth control pills], but now ... this!"

In the search for pregnancy, patients cling to the body, its rhythms, cycles, and fertility progressively acquiring new organisational value. At the doctor's appointment, the body returns via X-rays, ultrasounds, hormone therapy, and embryos in assisted reproduction; medical reports become testimonies of the body's interior, its fluids and depths.

In some cases, reaching a medical diagnosis may reduce anxiety. This was the case for Cristina and Juan: "The doctors told us he has varicocele[1]. We're more relaxed now. Something has already been found, and he accepts the problem in front of others," said Cristina. Juan nodded.

Undergoing clinical analyses without finding any organic issues had caused growing anxiety in this couple. It is the unpredictable body that generates anxiety. It is also common to find cases in which medical language is assimilated as their own, as in the following clinical vignette of Diana's case: "In March, I had an IUI[2] done, and his swim-up[3] results were 76%. Stimulation was with 8 milligrams and the other one was done with a higher dose ... I can't remember ..."

This new medical-like language reflects the patient's need to establish new bindings and "semantification" for the body through the doctor's words. It is also an attempt to master and bind the anxiety by using new codes, the doctor's words, which put words to what the couple does not know about their bodies. It shows a desire to understand the unpredictability of their bodies and to make it something familiar through medical terminology.

Piera Aulagnier (1979) points out that the body is an object of which we believe ourselves to be masters and owners. Nevertheless, it can also become the source or place from which suffering emerges, although the ego does not want it to or cannot anticipate it. Therefore, the body is rendered a frustrating object, alien to the ego: it undergoes medical examinations and is assisted in order to address the urgency of finding the cause of infertility somewhere inside.

In some cases, the journey through medical-technological treatments is highly sacrificial in essence, since it is associated with hostility towards a body that would not get pregnant. This hostility is observed in clinical work through the insistence of patients on carrying out further medical interventions, and changing professionals and also fertility centres in order to get pregnant, often without sufficient reflection. In these cases, the medical studies are aimed at modifying the bodies at all costs in order to access motherhood.

In other cases, difficulties in achieving pregnancy expose the need to modify the maternal ideal. This implies a narcissistic renunciation in the modification of the ideal of having a biological child, which broadens the paths to follow.

Up to this point, we have seen that complex body-mind bonds involve a multiplicity of psychic scenarios in women. We now show that they are also present in men.

The man's body

Male reproductive problems were not a topic of psychoanalytical research for a long time. Everything related to male infertility was surrounded by darkness that constituted a true "dark continent"[4]. Infertility experienced in a male body, though clinically observable, has been an under-researched area. Let us explore the case of Carlos and Adriana, who arrived at my consulting room a few days after receiving a diagnosis of azoospermia, that is, absence of sperm.

"The doctor was too honest. It was a bombshell … there is no sperm … who have I harmed? Did I wrong somebody?" said Carlos as he looked at Adriana.

"He is depressed. A a year ago he had another one done and it wasn't this bad. I've never seen him like this, he didn't go to work yesterday, he was sick all night, it started with pain in the back of the head. He cried."

From that moment on, Carlos began to suffer from gastrointestinal symptoms: diarrhoea, gastritis, and reflux. These symptoms were related to his inability to "digest" and "metabolise" this new reality. Apart from this, he started to work longer hours; he also lost his personal documents twice. These too were a way to give meaning to what he had lost: the genetic possibility of having his own biological children.

During the first stage of the analysis, Carlos and Adriana reported that they had not talked about this issue with their friends or family because of the embarrassment they felt when faced with the diagnosis of azoospermia. They were hesitant about how to move forward. They did not know whether to start with adoption papers or to undergo assisted fertilisation with semen from a donor. Their everyday life was impregnated with castration-related experiences associated with the impossibility of transmitting part of their genetic pool; this fact was highly meaningful for them since their families were traditional and blood ties were highly cathected.

The moratorium on research in male reproductive disorders is related to men's cultural role as genitors, providers, and those who uphold the law. In this sense, the ideals of virility, sexual potency, and fertility, all elements linked to the collective imaginary about men, have made male reproductive issues less visible. These ideals are examples of narcissised male functions (Hassoun, 1998).

Consequently, men with reproductive disorders tend to feel that part of their masculinity is being threatened, which often delays medical studies or analyses due to conscious or unconscious conflicts that emerge. In some cases, patients go through states of anguish and anxiety, since they feel that the medical studies are testing their sexual potency instead of their fertility. For instance, a spermogram[5] involves the recollection of semen via masturbation. This last element, though it may at first seem unimportant, may awaken such intense anxiety in some men that it becomes impossible to gather a sample. Sometimes there is a need for surgery, for example, after a diagnosis of varicocele[6].

Therefore, the diagnostic stage is marked by anxiety which, due to displacement, leads to different symptoms such as decreased sexual desire, insomnia, and fantasies about their overall health. Consequently, this may favour a tendency to give up the medical studies and the search for a child. Furthermore, it is not always easy for patients to share their concerns with their peers, since underlying sexist fantasies produce fears that they may be excluded from the circle of fertile and potent men.

Our current culture includes new perspectives on male fertility that lead away from the traditional androcentric ideals of masculinity. These habitual ideals used to mask, and in many cases still do, the suffering behind the impossibility of having children and what it means for each man.

The couple's body

As a couple journeys in their attempt to get pregnant[7], doctor's appointments and their vicissitudes become part of their history. The decision to consult, choosing a medical practitioner or a fertility clinic, implies the need to establish new agreements that serve as support for this new situation.

Undergoing studies, whether invasive or not, over a long period of time places the couple in a regressive situation, dependent on the functioning of their bodies. These bodies are suddenly studied, measured, and analysed, which is often experienced as if it were all an exam that had to be passed. However, there is nothing more unpredictable than our bodies. Who can anticipate its movements, the changes in its fluids, and its depths?

On this journey through medical appointments, couples pour out their expectations, fears, and desires. Therefore, transference with the doctor or the medical team is intensely cathected in the expectation that the fertility of their bodies will receive care.

At this stage, many couples have to let go of the idea of the "scheduled child," supposed to arrive once the relationship has strengthened, the couple settled into a house, having interrupted the use of contraceptive methods in order to begin the search for a child.

When the "scheduled" pregnancy does not occur, people lose the illusion of control over their bodies, their plans, and their projects. Everything is brought to a halt and they can no longer picture their lives as they used to. Therefore, their belief in the natural quality of biological processes related to their reproductive capacities crumbles, dragging the ideal of control down with it.

We know that the idea of planned parenthood grew stronger thanks to the advent of oral contraception in the 1960s and reproductive technology in the 1980s. Yet when difficulties arise, the body is no longer seen as something that can be predicted or controlled. Given the expectations of a natural pregnancy and the promise of control over the bodily functions, infertility requires a new space to be thought out both at an individual level and at the level of links.

A portion of their intimacy is no longer part of their private life. In medical consultations, bodies become visible through sonograms, X-rays, and analyses that report their functioning.

Some people share this issue with friends and family, whereas others reserve it as a topic to be discussed only in their intimacy. The anxiety of airing the issue sometimes leads them into a period of isolation. Consequently, they stop meeting their family or friends who have children since they experience anxiety and want to avoid talking about the problem, as was the case with Gabriel and Ana:

> I feel so-so. It's this concrete reality of ours. The test showed zero sperm, so did the other one I had, zero. I don't know, if I can't have children she should be free. I respect her process but it's the woman who suffers

Anna said, "I don't agree. I think it's a two-way street ... I need his support!"

This couple began their analysis after many medical consultations that confirmed Gabriel's diagnosis. In the session, he explained that he had undergone surgery in childhood because his testicles had not descended[8], but he'd never thought it could have consequences on his fertility.

Gabriel said, "Everything looks black or white for me now, I can't see any grey, Why me? If I'd known about this before, I don't know if I would have married. A child of one's own is something you long for, something you feel. You can see yourself projected in your children, I have no one to look at! I feel as if there were a huge wall and I can't jump over it. I feel no one can help me. Why, God, have you forsaken me?"

This session developed in an atmosphere of great anxiety. The diagnosis of azoospermia not only reactivated Gabriel's castration anxiety but also led to the experience of rupture of the generational chain. His despair showed how important blood ties were for him and his need for filiation, for belonging, and for being someone's son and someone's father. Gabriel often expressed that he felt not only pain but also embarrassment after the diagnosis. At the same time, Ana developed organic symptoms due to this situation. She had acute gastritis and then suffered a false appendicitis, which led her to be hospitalised and in observation for several days.

Gabriel's suffering body echoed in Ana's body in the manner of an identifying couvade[9] in which she also fell ill to accompany him in a body-to-body mirror.

As the analysis moved forward, a dilemma arose: whether to set out on a journey towards adoption or resort to sperm donation from a sperm bank. Having a life without children was not a possibility in their life project.

The most difficult task for this couple was to start talking about the subject and to enter this unknown territory that sometimes presents, in Freudian terms, "uncanny" scenarios in which the familiar is somehow strange[9] (Freud, 1919). Thus, Gabriel began by asking some questions that had been silenced during his childhood: why did his parents never say anything? Didn't they know about the consequences? Didn't the doctor give them enough information? Or maybe they knew and didn't want to or perhaps didn't dare to tell him. However, Gabriel did not want to talk about these questions with his parents due to his intense ambivalence towards them. Above all, he did not want to talk to them because he needed to avoid losing any support.

Throughout the analysis, the place of their bodies in the couple's history and their families was present. Such was the universe of meanings worked through.

We may find different clinical scenarios. Lack of pregnancy frequently begins to cast its shadow over the course of several months, as Raquel said. "We stopped using protection two years ago. In the beginning I was more relaxed. Now I'm not, I see a pregnant woman and I get upset. I don't know, when I have my period, I fall apart."

Oral contraception and the use of reproductive techniques establish a radical separation between reproduction and sexual life. Trying to conceive frequently causes interest for sexual life to wane, whereas the desire, expectation, and wait for a pregnancy predominate. In this context, couples witness a change when they go through psychic modifications as they confirm that their desires and fantasies are fading away. The different clinical cases presented so far show the multiplicity of meanings these problems entail.

In many cases, we observe that initial longing for a child gradually becomes a distressing and sometimes paralysing situation. Whether overt or covert, these depressive states accompany the decrease in sexual desire.[10] The passion in the sexuality that initiates the search for pregnancy tends to lose vitality. The possibility of pregnancy is hyper-cathected and sexuality is relegated to the background: the central concern is to get pregnant.

There may be cases that present difficulties in their sexual life prior to the search for a pregnancy. They seek fertility assistance, but doctors discover that it is the couple's sexual life that is affecting conception, apart from other factors at play. These difficulties may be overlooked at a medical consultation, obvious as they may seem. Therefore, couples initiate a series of tests although it is precisely their sex life that lies at the root of infertility.

Changes in the couple's sexual desire may also be accompanied by other aspects of their sexual life. In the case of women, vaginismus and dyspareunia hinder sex life and pleasure and may also entail difficulties or inhibitions in seeking medical assistance. In men, instances of erectile dysfunction or premature ejaculation may sometimes be discovered in the face of certain medical tests.

Love and sexual encounters may also be hindered by the couple's daily schedule. One may work at night and the other during the day, or they may work rotating shifts throughout the month. Janine Puget and Isidoro Berenstein (1992) suggest that the couple's everyday life is one of the parameters to consider in couple therapy. Another parameter is the couple's shared life project, in which the arrival of children is often a priority. The third parameter is their sexual life, which is subordinated to reproduction in the contexts discussed here. Finally, the authors propose taking into account the monogamous tendency together with parameters of fidelity.

It is therefore evident that many aspects of the couple's life are involved in the search for pregnancy. Therefore, it is vital to adopt an approach that takes links into account, since the couple's and the individuals' desires and projects may be eclipsed by trying to conceive.

There tend to be two cycles of everyday life from the emotional point of view. During the first part of the monthly cycle, expectations and spirits are high, and thus sexuality responds actively. However, after the ovulatory peak in the second part of the cycle, there is anxiety, and sexuality declines as the wait for a result sets in. Finally, women may experience menstruation as a loss. This emotional fluctuation is described as the *emotional roller coaster* of sexual desire in cases of infertility (Martin, 1994).

Furthermore, whenever doctors suggest specific days and times for sexual relations, they may become mechanical. As a consequence, desire and spontaneity decrease and couples may fall into apathy.

Finally, another element worth considering in the analysis is the doctor as a third party in intimacy. There are no longer only two people, but three or more if a medical team is involved. In this relationship, ambivalent feelings of trust and distrust, idealisation and denigration, and hope and despair develop.

The use of complex assisted reproductive technology, in which fertilisation is extracorporeal since it takes place in a laboratory, entails an additional psychic effort for the couple, since this deeply emotional process is shared with the doctor or the medical team. In these cases, the separation between sexual and reproductive life is total. Sex life is completely separated from reproductive life: conception is achieved outside the body and the embryo only nests in it. Fantasies of passivity grow, and it becomes evident that the fertility of the couple is only possible through medical assistance. Thus, fantasies of shared parenthood are established.

When all these problems cause great anxiety, they may affect the couple's affective closeness both at the emotional and the sexual level. This journey demands intense physical and psychic effort from the couple and each of the partners.

In the light of the reproductive-related difficulties facing these couples, it is important for them to rescue their capacity to reproduce but also to think: about whether to move forward or to say, "Enough." It is true that nowadays it is difficult for a couple to consider that they have tried everything. Every scientific breakthrough gives them new hope and also makes it difficult for them to stop: it seems that there is always something else to try. In the clinic, we can see how difficult it is to leave hard reality behind and think about how to move forward. The desire for a child peremptorily imposes itself so that it prevents couples from ceasing to try. Sometimes they face a new type of suffering; for example, when a couple cannot undergo a given treatment and they experience it as yet another failure.

In conclusion, sexual life and reproductive life in patients with infertility difficulties are split and drift apart into two separate channels. This may produce short- or long-term effects on the relationship. For this reason, a psychoanalytic approach that focuses on the relationship is essential.

From a clinical point of view, it is important to bear in mind the peremptory nature of these consultations, but also to aim at the recovery of sensuality and sexuality along this journey.

Transparent bodies into technology

Social representations assign a particular symbolism to bodies within societies. Knowledge about the body is tributary to a culture that defines its subjects. Images of bodies and their interior have been amplified and are easily accessible for us thanks to technological advances. For example, gametes (ovum and spermatozoa) are measured in microns, yet they can be seen and manipulated. Therefore, the reproductive system holds almost no secrets for the human eye.

A certain opacity in regard to the body has covered it across centuries (Le Breton, 1995). However, bodies have now become transparent thanks to the amplification of otherwise inaccessible images via technology. Images and transparency constitute the body's figurability nowadays, when we are able to see beyond perception and "imaginarise" the parts that are gestating new life.

As a result, a different bodily nature emerges. Apart from the combination of fluids, cells, and organs, *transparent bodies* that hold no secrets appear. Everything is visible and possible in the current imaginary: motherhood in the woman's 20s, 40s, or 60s.

We return to the image. The subject and the image share a certain alienation from the body: they belong to the body's ego, yet they are an object. Sonograms, X-rays, and pictures of embryos are flat, bi-dimensional pictures: the projection of the body on a surface. These pictures reflect the body and work as a scaffold to bind and represent the unknown interiority. In every history, medical discourse is built through a file full of tests, words, and images. The protagonists may be unaware of them, but the pictures are still a reflection of their bodies.

Therefore, these images create a new narrative of the body. Its nature is different and, in some cases, the body is half one's own and half someone else's as in instances of surrogacy: when a woman gestates a baby for another. As Ehrensaft (2018) notes, surrogacy includes women and men, gender diversity, genetic diversity via gamete donation, and diversity in wombs of the women carrying the pregnancies. The combination of bodies, gametes, and fluids in surrogacy is diversified on a case-by-case basis. Another example is the embryos created with the father's genetic material, but not with the surrogate's genetic material.

The transparency and multiplicity of the bodies evoke the image of a "Medusa's head." In these contexts, multiplicity is an effect of castration or the lack thereof. These techniques seem to conceal an underlying message: "This body is not infertile. It is fertile."

The idea of a body that is "technologically complete" is present. The imaginary of a transparent and adaptable body introduces new narratives related to problems concerning the psychic inscriptions of these experiences. In other words, they are linked to the process of working through the rupture in the means of conception and the imaginary related to a transparent and predictable body.

Extracorporeal fertilisation (the *in vitro* procedure in a laboratory) introduces a new element: since the embryonic gestations take place there, the doctors acquire the gestational function. This is an unprecedented experience for couples, since they can "see" the embryos: they can zoom in on the image; they can take photos. All these experiences are inscribed as something new.

Furthermore, these new fertilisation techniques differ significantly from the way their parents, grandparents, and previous generations conceived. Hence, the experience adopts a "disturbing strangeness" that stems from a rupture in the traditional method of conception. This "uncanny" situation should be put into words in order to discover what it evokes in each subject. The scenario is more complex when another person's genetic material is involved as in cases of donation of gametes (ovum or spermatozoa), surrogate and deferred motherhood, among other examples. How can we "imaginarise" the gestation of these embryos that come from this new architecture of a body whose transparency appears to reveal all its secrets?

We analysts should consider the psychic impact of these new technologies given the wide range of meanings to these new parenthoods.

However, analysts may sustain prejudices, values, or ethical issues in regard to these techniques. We belong to the "pre-test-tube generation." Consequently, it is strange for the analyst to "imaginarise" body parts in another person's body creating life.

We are the first generation in human history to deal with extracorporeal fertilisation. The uncanny disturbing strangeness that we face forces us to reflect on procreation as something separate from sexuality. It also leads us to reflect on the difference that technology establishes in what was once sacredly preserved for oneself.

The body in transference

The body reintroduces something barely related to the biological body into the analytic relation. However, the subject-analyst relation deals with the biological aspect in the first place.

In this respect, Cain (1994) proposes to consider that the body defines an inside, an outside, and also transit routes. Although disturbance may be on the outside (the wrappings), the inside and the roads connecting interior and exterior are also affected.

Cain also suggests bearing in mind that an illness, whichever it may be, becomes the support for a fundamental bond with another person. Finally, the symptom, whichever it may be, involves phantasmatic activity that should be taken into consideration. He points out that psychoanalysis reintroduces the body through the analytic process.

In the context of reproductive disorders, concrete elements impregnate the sessions: figures, medical tests, and recurrent surgeries. Thus, the bond with the body develops during the analysis. Expectations for the future and the incessant and peremptory search for pregnancy acquire a specific meaning and exert force in the analysis. The intrapsychic path that orders that there "must" be a pregnancy is central to this process. This imperative is thus transferred into the analytical relation: the analysis is seen as "fertilisation" that must work inside the body to render it fertile.

I believe it is now necessary to establish a difference given that the same word does not always mean the same. It is not a question of anxiety stemming from the phantasy of infertility of a patient in analysis, but of anxiety experienced by a person who is sterile or infertile. Even though we may say that anxiety is an objectless fear, we should discern the patient's anxiety whose object is the patient's own reality of sterility. Something of the real body is present in transference.

Piera Aulagnier (1979) explains that the real body and the mental representation of our body confront one another in these situations. By means of psychic work, the analytical process is at the intersection in which the real body and its mental representation meet. There, it operates at the heart of peremptory and narcissistic urgency usually found in the sessions. The questions that enable analytical work will acquire a fertilising function as it develops the complex relations between the mental representation of the body and the real body.

The child that has not arrived: Clinical cases of mourning

In one session, Daniela cried out, "I can't stand seeing pregnant women. The city is full of them. I can't stand seeing them!" This clipped view of reality reflects the contents of her mind. In her eyes, the world is full of pregnant women, which contrasts with her pregnancy that does not occur. The *pregnant women* signifier is built around a mute witness of something missing. It is experienced as a narcissistic wound due to the impossibility of achieving the pregnancy.

The child to come, a love object not found in the present, lives in her mind as a loss referring to an unattained ideal. It also points to mourning due to her impossibility to procreate. In a manner of speaking, castration is therefore represented by the everyday experience of not being pregnant. Let us remember that Freud (1917) defines *mourning* as the reaction to losing a loved one, an abstraction that stands in for them, such as homeland, freedom, or an ideal. He describes the grieving nature of mourning as the genuine reaction towards loss.

Let us focus on mourning, its grieving affect, and depressive states as objects of analysis in this section. They are all recurring clinical manifestations in consultations about infertility which impregnate the emotional atmosphere of the analysis.

When a patient is referred to a psychoanalyst, the inner workings of the body or the location of disorders in reproductive organs are no longer the focal point. It is about being able to assign new meanings to their experiences. Thus, analytical listening aims at helping the patient to abandon the density of anatomy: to move from the body to words and to transform infertility into a question.

Throughout the analysis, patients develop their anxiety, often silenced in everyday life while inhabiting their minds with toxic effects. In these cases, we often encounter mourning processes with particular features that are not reactions to the loss of a real object. What is worse, no mourning ritual exists for the absence of a pregnancy month after month.

Therefore, there is a double inscription in this mourning process: in the body and in the mind. The object cannot yet be found in reality and what was lost is not a loved person but a child to be loved.

Day after day and month after month, patients reveal expectations projected onto the treatment to be undergone the following month or the following year. How can we categorise this new absent object of love that condenses multiple meanings? In psychoanalysis, we know that a child is an object narcissistically invested as an extension of the self.

David Nasio (1996) defines mourning as a task with its own time. It fundamentally depends on the love experience that each subject had with the lost object. Nasio adds that the pain stems from the intensity of the representations of the loved object, which now lack the support of the image the object once gave in return. In cases of infertility, the longed-for child emerges as an imaginary support. Therefore, a bond forms between the absent child and the monthly grief after again discovering its absence.

Persistence is easily observable when patients share their feelings and experiences related to infertility in clinical work. Histories always revolve around the same topics: tests they are undergoing, their results, and how long they have been on this journey. The scene repeats itself as a traumatic situation that attempts to be rewritten, driven by repetition compulsion. For many couples, this pilgrimage becomes the one and only topic due to the urgency of the treatments, tests, and results.

Constant talk about the same problem, repetitive thoughts about treatments, and the time that has passed are present in everyday life. Analytical work aims at transforming psychic pain into tolerable suffering, facilitating the mourning process by which the patient will enable other desires. However, in many cases, the pain does not evolve to be worked through, but remains as an open wound. It persists throughout fertility treatments and gives rise to depressive states of varying intensity. These are sometimes manifested in aggressive feelings towards those closest to them and libidinal withdrawal and hopelessness.

Bleichmar (1991) describes depression as showing sadness, psychomotor retardation, and self-reproach as clinical features; also a pessimistic view of life and an affective state of sadness. He adds that the patient's fixed desire seems to be unattainable; this is the central thought of patients with depression, regardless of the ways it manifests itself.

For most patients, the depressive states are periodic and brief; however, for other patients, they accompany the entire process. The situation is more complex if we consider that the conscious desire for a child may conceal unconscious rejection, or strong ambivalence, towards motherhood or fatherhood.

The search for a child might mask a depression of a different nature. It is essential to distinguish depressive states caused by the distress produced by infertility from depression caused by previous mourning left unspoken or not worked through, masked by the search for a child. In these cases, the child is intended to fill the place of the lost object. Hence, depressive states are reinforced by preceding mourning. Therefore, the compulsive demand for a child may be understood as a symptom of pathological mourning.

In the following clinical vignette, the patient's consultation for infertility masked unresolved mourning.

Unresolved mourning

Paula (34) and Martín (36) came to analysis after four years' trying to achieve a pregnancy by different means. They had gone through a range of medical tests and several unsuccessful fertility treatments. The doctor who referred them had dismissed any significant organic factors that would affect the couple's fertility. Therefore, he considered that the couple should not continue undergoing medical treatments but instead ask for couple's psychoanalytic therapy.

They talked very little about their parental families in initial interviews. The focus revolved around infertility.

Paula once said, "I had the insemination done yesterday, so this week I'll be more relaxed. The only issue is that I'm sick of getting so many injections, but it's my only option. Martin tried giving me the injections this month and he did it."

A significant element in Paula's story was her father's death some months before their wedding. She later corrected herself and explained in an unemotional tone of voice that he had committed suicide.

Paula and Martín, showing little capacity for historicising themselves, used a rather evacuative discourse attached to concrete facts about the treatments. This element became important later in view of the traumatic situation that defined it: the trauma operated by unbinding.

"We are moving forward," said Martín, "but we are in the final stretch. After this, there is nothing else. We have to continue with the in vitro thing and then adoption as a long term possibility." He then continued, "The fact that we are healthy and we go on and on and on … I think we'll get tired at some point. We'll reach saturation and say: we've done so much; we shouldn't do anything else."

"You get the same thing every month," said Paula, "In 28 days it all starts again.[11] It's kind of a habit …"

"Yes," Martín agreed, "it's this wheel that keeps spinning every month. One cycle finishes and then another one starts. That's the way we see it at the moment. I think it's pretty much like that."

Whenever the emotional atmosphere might have enabled asking questions and detaching from concrete elements, they displayed resistance. It consequently deprived their discourse of affection and led the conversation back to the treatments.

As the analysis advanced, remnants of Paula's father's suicide began to surface like debris from a shipwreck, regardless of the silence about their close family. This silence, I started to understand, was a sort of protection from returning to a scene they had been escaping.

They once arrived a few minutes late due to a traffic jam. At the start of that session, Paula said, "I was driving, and he kept saying 'Get into the lane; because if you stop, everyone but you will get in'."

It was her inability to stop this evacuative and quasi-operational modality. She was talking about strong resistance to a different, dormant, and extremely dangerous topic: "everyone is getting in." Is every pain getting in at the same time?

This inability continued in later sessions. It was difficult to get into that particular lane of circulation of affects and thoughts.

"Would you say that all this search for a child has in any way modified how the two of you used to be, I mean looking backwards?" said the analyst.

"No, not at all," Martin replied.

"No, not at all. We've always been there for each other. When one of us is down, the other tries to lift them up," Paula said.

"This situation didn't cause any problems. It didn't wear us out," Martin said.

Finally, after some time, the problem of Paula's father's suicide emerged. Paula told me her father had a bad temper, it was difficult to anticipate his reactions, and he was violent. By the end of the session, we managed to tie the couple's infertility to Paula's father's suicide:

> "Have you ever considered that this issue could be linked to something else?" the analyst asked and added, "we sometimes associate some problems with other issues, strange as it may seem. Maybe this is related to your difficulty in having children."

"Everyone tells me that what happened to my dad may have affected me indirectly," Paula answered.

"Is that what they say or what you think?" the analyst asked.

"I'm not sure whether it has affected me or not. Martín's told me the same thing thousands of times, and so has my mum" answered Paula. "They tell me, there must be something in you because of what happened to your father. The thing is, at the moment my dad died, killed himself, I couldn't react, I didn't take in the situation. I didn't go into the funeral wake to see him."

At that moment, in the countertransference, I was surprised by the natural way she said this. It was also the first time she had ever mentioned that experience in the analytical process. It was as if she had lifted the veil of the relation between her father's traumatic death and infertility. This was a fragment of their story whose elements allowed us to work through this pathological mourning: a depression incarnated in their infertile bodies.

The session continued.

"The question is why he did it," Martin said, "if it was vengeance for our wedding."

"Vengeance?" asked the analyst.

"He used to say he wasn't going to be at our wedding. So since he said that ... I don't know if she took it in. I don't know," Martín said. He hesitated since it was difficult for him to find the right words to express himself.

> I don't know how she took what he said to her. He used to say that we were too busy with our own things and were leaving him aside. He said that we didn't care about what he was going through (Martín points out that Paula's father was depressed) and that we were busy planning our wedding.

"My mom asked me, 'but are we having the party anyway?' and I said I wanted to have the party anyway; and she would say 'but there's going to be music and we're going to dance ....'"

Following Paula's ideas, we may add: are we going to live? Are we going to have children? Are we going to think about ourselves?

It was Martín who embodied nostalgia: "Her father would have helped us so much if he were here."

The suicide crystallised an idealised image of a strong man who was also feared given his unpredictable and violent reactions: "I was terrified of my father. When he was angry, he could be very aggressive."

Her father's suicide triggered pathological mourning that fixed the couple onto a compulsive search for a child; a barren search since the forces at work in conjugal sterility were linked to the inability to mourn. They were both children who had survived a traumatic experience.

Thanks to the difficult and painful development of this mourning process, Paula shared the news of her pregnancy sometime afterwards. It was unnecessary to mourn this absent father forever.

The analytical work aided the couple to break away from the thanatic and repetitive cycles. As a result, they could work through the issue and continued throughout her pregnancy and the birth of their child. What had never been inscribed had at last been given some room in their history. They could think about it without experiencing the pain and fear of it being razed. Conjugal infertility was a symptom of depression. Analytical work allowed this symptom to become the starting point for working through the mourning of her father's tragic death.

As mentioned above, the imaginary child replaces the lost object and is also a means to avoid the painful mourning process for the loss of the real object. In other words, when patients are going through pathological mourning that cannot be worked through, they mourn the absence of a child instead of mourning the lost object.

In conclusion, couples who seek help in relation to reproductive disorders deal with different clinical scenarios that sometimes encompass mourning or depressive states of varying intensity. Only by adopting a new perspective in analytical work is it possible to work through these experiences. Just as Freud, S. (1873–1939) wrote to Marta Bernays: it is not possible to enjoy the present if we do not understand it or if we do not understand the past[12].

Permanent infertility

Although there are different means of achieving a pregnancy in the field of assisted reproductive technology, the presence of a biological impossibility to conceive constitutes a narcissistic wound that requires psychic processing. Patients usually approach analysis after being diagnosed with azoospermia in men or early menopause in women. Their working through this impossibility to transmit their genetic pool is unique in each analysis regardless of available therapeutic alternatives. In cases of azoospermia in men, patients may resort to sperm banks, whereas in cases of early menopause in women, ovum or embryo donation is an alternative[13].

The diagnosis of permanent infertility due to azoospermia operated as a traumatic element for Alberto and Liliana.

Alberto said,

> "We've been thinking non-stop for a week about what the doctor told us ... we'll have to adopt or look for a donor to have a child ... I would never have imagined anything like this. All my siblings have children and I can't! We feel really bad about all this ..." Liliana stares at him and cries in silence.

In the context of permanent infertility, there may be uterine malformations or absence of the uterus in women. Surrogate motherhood has been an alternative for gestation in these cases since the 1970s, however controversial it may be in ethical and legislative respects.

I would like to share a brief clinical vignette. Many years ago, the gynaecology department at Maternidad Sardá [Sardá Mothers and Children's Hospital] requested an inter-consultation with the department of psychopathology for a 22-year-old patient who had had an emergency hysterectomy[14].

After this woman was discharged, her husband was standing in the corridor holding her bags and waiting to leave. Meanwhile, a pale young woman with long hair was in the general ward, still wrapped in a hospital gown as if she were unable to move. It was a scene replete with desolation.

As the analyst said goodbye, she said to her, "Yes, you had your uterus surgically removed, but no one removed your desire to become a mother." Some years later, in a non-professional context, a young woman the analyst did not recognise approached her. This woman asked her if she was a doctor and reminded her of the episode described above. Finally, the woman said: "Doctor, I have a child. I adopted a girl." The analyst says that she still feels moved by this memory[15].

In this clinical vignette, the patient had to deal with permanent infertility as she had had a hysterectomy. She went on a journey to work through her impossibility to get pregnant and embarked on the trip to adoption. It is clear that the analyst's intervention left a mark on this woman's life.

In conclusion, the mourning process in cases of permanent infertility may encounter obstacles to accepting this new geography of the body. It implies accepting a body image that is different from the image previously held. In this clinical vignette, the patient's working through enabled her to access motherhood. Just as her analyst had pointed out, it was her capacity to conceive biologically that had been altered, but her desire to become a mother was intact.

Up to this point, we have discussed mourning in cases of irreversible diagnoses. However, we may also encounter cases in which difficulties to conceive may be treated via restorative and non-substitutive treatments. In the next section, I share a clinical case in which the impossibility for conceiving took a troubled path.

Transitory infertility[16]

Marcela (38) and Julian (39) had been married for eight years, and Marcela had a 15-year-old son from a previous marriage. After spending their lives together for some time, they shared a desire to have a child. However, after some years with no pregnancy, they made their first medical consultations. During this journey, Marcela underwent two laparoscopic surgeries[17] due to endometriosis[18], three procedures of intrauterine insemination[19], and an in vitro fertilisation[20].

During analysis, Marcela said that she wanted to be a mother again and *give Julián a child*. She was concerned about the passing of time and signs of it running out, fully aware of her *biological clock*. The urgency when she consulted was to attempt a new assisted fertility treatment while experiencing discomfort in a relationship inhabited by quarrels.

Analytical work experienced initial difficulties and resistance in relation to the frequency of sessions. The setting required at least two sessions a week. Although she accepted this, Marcela felt it was too intense. In the first stage of the analysis, the topics were exhaustion and pain stemming from the physical and psychic efforts she had made during the surgical interventions, the medical tests, and, above all, from expectations that were not met. She had experienced all this in silence. Talking about it or even recalling the experiences in analysis involved *bringing everything back to life*, connecting again with anxiety. It involved going through the commotion caused by a body that had become the source of intense unpleasure.

This ambivalence at the onset of analysis was related to a paradox: wanting to be listened to while being unable to talk. Marcela began to talk about her relationship with her mother, who would leave her alone in moments of crisis. This was repeated in transference when she decided to undergo another assisted reproduction treatment during the summer when her analyst was on holiday. It was repetition compulsion: she was re-experiencing abandonment, now by her analyst, who was in the position of the mother who abandoned her in crises. When sessions resumed after the vacation, she told me that the fertility treatment had been unsuccessful.

Marcela said,

> It went badly. It didn't work. 14 days waiting for the results ... On Saturday, I just snapped. First, I checked my hormone levels and they were low, maybe I was pregnant! But two days later, I checked again and no, there was no pregnancy. The same thing happened again.

She continued, "We took some days off to travel. We got along really well there, we relaxed. But I don't know, we've been having problems since we got back ... I told him I felt he was punishing me and he answered that I'm being nasty and I frown at him."

This new unsuccessful treatment reactivated mourning from all her previous treatments that Marcela found really difficult and painful to work through. Moreover, there were confrontations and arguments between the couple.

At this stage of her analysis, Marcela shared her anxiety about the constant confrontation with Julián. This unsuccessful pregnancy resulted in complex mourning that had a direct impact on the marital link.

"He tells me 'you're destructive and so ill-disposed.' I don't know, everything is falling apart," she said.

There was intense aggression in her link with Julián; discomfort and incomprehension grew in Marcela. As a consequence, the situation became extremely critical, and the idea of a break-up was raised.

Marcela had two episodes of menstrual bleeding between her periods at this stage. She experienced this situation as discomfort placed in her body through bleeding. This was also an expression of her pain at not being able to mourn the pregnancy with Julián. This silent mourning in the couple was transformed into hostility. Questions about the future arose.

The language of her body led her to wonder about the bleedings: there were two bleedings and also two assisted reproduction treatments. They were the children who could not arrive.

"I had an argument with Julián on Sunday. I was very upset," she said.

The analyst said, "Complaints and reproaches have become a habit. Is it a way of punishing yourself for not having achieved a pregnancy?"

Marcela said, "He is carrying a burden and I feel bad, too. He is going through his things and I don't ask him about anything. We're distant and are both going through our individual issues. He changed cars, bought a brand new car, and I didn't say a thing ... On Tuesday, I woke up feeling bad, feeling down."

"There's a way of arguing set up in your relationship, but we know that sadness and pain is behind it. You can fight, but you can't cry together," said the analyst.

"It's that he gets angry ... I don't know," she said. "In fact, with the pregnancy ...(silence) "I still have four embryos left. I don't know, this has devastated me."

Marcela was overwhelmed by the situation. Julián displaced his castration anxiety onto buying a brand new car, a substitute for something he could not actually have.

In this context, Marcela took a melancholic path and considered leaving Julián so that he could have children with another woman. It was a self-imposed punishment for not being able to give him a child. She felt responsible for this failure and therefore guilty, surrendering to suffering.

In this couple, the difficulties of working through the mourning of a failed pregnancy, which reactivated other losses, gave the floor to bodily language in the form of repetitive symptoms: gastrointestinal disorders in Julián and bleeding in Marcela.

Their constant quarrelling expressed a particular mode of dealing with mourning that seemed to become pathological, since they tolerated aggression despite the shared discomfort. They were unable to share the sadness and pain that arose from the failure of the treatments. As a consequence, the couple's link underwent a movement in which the fighting drove them further apart, disconnecting them from the loving aspects that once brought them together. It was a melancholic journey in which the lost child-object has cast its shadow over their link.

In the light of this case, it is possible to reflect on clinical work with couples who undergo assisted reproduction treatments due to transitory infertility. Although medical therapy is available to them, their journey may still be complex. For some couples, as for Marcela and Julián, these experiences invade much of the couple's love history. They involve a process of mourning and transformation or a process of repetition. Patients need to face losing their reproductive capacity for carrying their child in their womb. Despite technological advances and the couple's determination, something is taken away from the couple, blocking the opening of other roads of access to parenthood.

In conclusion, mourning in these cases becomes a never-ending process, since the promise of future fertility always renews hope in a new treatment to finally achieve a pregnancy that will result in the arrival of a child. The problem lies in determining the limit of these hopefulness-hopelessness cycles, mainly because these journeys leave a mark in the lives of couples and inside both bodies.

When fertility treatments are unsuccessful and result in no pregnancy, couples wonder: when can we say "enough"?

Enigmatic infertility

María is a patient I saw several years ago. She came to the consultation after being diagnosed by her doctor as infertile without any apparent cause. This analysis was a place of changes not only in the patient, but also demanded that I as her analyst reconsider things in several circumstances and prioritise one subject over another issue, no less important.

She was late for her first interview, arriving in a state of anxiety and anguish. She was a 30-year-old woman with a neat appearance, very tidy. The way she was dressed caught my attention because of the many details.

The first thing she mentioned, besides the problem, was: "I'm not getting pregnant," and her "nerves"—which I translated as her enormous anxiety. She asked me for something, some medicine to calm her down. She was nearly on the edge of tears. I explained that I couldn't medicate her and proposed that we think together about what was going on.

She said she gets depressed with every menstruation and is willing to do whatever is needed to achieve a pregnancy. She began to tell how in the first years of her sexual life she was "obsessed" with the fear of getting pregnant and monitored the arrival of each period on time. During this period, of her adolescence, she did get pregnant more than once and decided to have abortions because "the conditions to have a child were not given. I lived with my mother."

She said she had been seeking a pregnancy for over three years, adding an important event: her mother's death a few months earlier.

María said, "With Raúl we've known each other for 16 years. We moved in together. At first we used birth control pills so we wouldn't get pregnant because we were living at my mother-in-law's. But it's been three years since we haven't taken them, because we have a house of our own."

The analyst asked, "When did you start to feel more 'nervous'?"

María said, "Well … actually, especially since my mom passed away … five months ago."

"How did she pass away?" the analyst asked.

María replied, "Vaginal cancer. (weeping silently) … Left me empty. I used to be almost her mother, she was so weak. Daddy died 11 years ago of cirrhosis. They were separated … I do have a brother, but he is on my mother's side … He depended on me. We didn't really get on with that man (referring to the stepfather)."

Later in the session: "Everything was in agreement between my husband and me. But now I'm upset with him."

"All in agreement …?" the analyst asked.

"He wants to have a child, I'm in doubt. I missed four abortions … I got pregnant when I was 18, and had no choice, but he didn't want to, so I told him: Raúl, I can't live like this, by myself, with a child, with my mother."

The sentence "I missed four abortions" is registered this way in material, but I am not sure if it was formulated this way or if it was a condensation when taking notes. My impression was that she was not very impressed by our first encounter. She was hoping I would give her something, maybe a pill. On the other hand, this was her first "psychological" experience, so she probably arrived with a "medical model," seeking a "remedy."

María talked about her ambivalence about whether to have a child with Raúl or not. Ambivalence is a very common issue in consultations of women seeking a pregnancy. Motherhood is often presented in conflict with other female desires or projects in opposition or that constitute obstacles. These include, for instance, work or maternity, or not having a partner and deciding to have a child, or the age of women who begin their search for pregnancy later in life. Different conflicts regarding the desire for a child are present when seeking a pregnancy.

In María's case, in this first interview, her conflictive relationship with Raúl is present. She is "willing to do whatever is needed" to get pregnant despite her doubts. It comes across as if she has decided to ignore her doubts, perhaps because she is not willing to seriously question the relationship and/or she is trying to please Raúl. Many questions emerged after the first encounter with María.

She also arrived late and restless to the second interview. She said she had been "a little bit less nervous," but complained of intense pain in the "mouth" of the stomach. When talking about the mouth of the stomach, she touches herself and points at the place.

She wanted to see a doctor because she felt bad. She spoke about her diet and attempted to discover some connection between her eating and those pains, searching for the reason for her distress somewhere. She did not speak much about her parents. Her mother was very submissive and weak, her father was an alcoholic and violent, and she had little memory of him. They separated when she was five years old. After the separation, her mother began a new relationship from which her brother was born. She rarely saw her father. He died when María was 18 years old.

Always very close to her mother, she never got along with her stepfather. At the moment of the consultation, her brother was 22 years old, in a relationship, and had a daughter who was a few months old.

She had met Raúl in her teens at the age of 14. The "unexpected" pregnancies that ended in abortions were between 18 and 21 years of age. She did not remember the dates accurately but she was living with her mother. At 24, they moved together into Raúl's mother's house and began to seek a pregnancy only when they moved out on their own.

It seemed to me that the reason for the consultation, rather than infertility, was the mourning for her mother, and because of the intense emotional link she had with her, she now wanted to re-create it with a child. I also noticed her mother's vaginal cancer (uterus cancer?); the vagina/womb was associated with death, the lack of life through infertility. The questions that came up in the first period of analysis were marked by the impossibility of having children, stomach discomfort, and her almost permanent anxiety.

During one session in the second month, while she talked about the tests being done, when referring to other medical practices, she said:

M: I had an operation on my ankle.
A: Why did you have the operation?
M: I had a fracture of my tibia and fibula.
A: Did you have an accident? (I don't understand why I'm asking such a direct question, but it was already spoken.)
M: ...No ... (silence) Raúl hit me, so I fell.
A: Raúl hits you ...
M: ... from time to time ... Because of arguments ... (with some embarrassment). However, I had a problem in an ear and he didn't hit me anymore.
A: A problem in an ear?
M: He was jealous because I'd been chatting with a friend. He smacked me in the face and cuffed my ear, so I said, "You made me deaf! When I got checked out, I found out that my ear was pierced ...
A: You lost your sense of hearing in that ear ...
M: I'm very annoyed ... I was pretending. I didn't want to show my mother anything. She was very tense, like she had never grown up.

I felt very shocked by the unexpectedness of this story and by María's ambivalence about including or excluding the subject of conjugal violence. María is a battered woman. I could almost say that we stumbled upon this issue in the session, which she related with modesty. How to continue working, since this revelation is not only a "topic" but a question to explore.

She always talked about the different studies and laboratory results ordered by the medical team; the surgery was several years ago. Her body, which initially presented an "enigmatic infertility," is now also a battered body.

In this session, an unexpected conjugal issue emerged: physical violence. However, María stood by her "infertility," anchored in that subject, not registering the violence as something "to be treated."

It was a crucial session in which she was able to talk about and put words to physical violence, a subject she had never discussed with her mother or any of her friends. Violence in this sense operates by unbinding: it is common for patients to hide it or to disguise their wounds.

In the following session, she arrived punctually and began to talk about her work.

M: I'm a dressmaker. I was looking for work as a dressmaker to leave the job I have. So, I'm going to see what I'm going to do.

(I associate this information with the details of her clothes which had drawn my attention in the first session. Her clothes as wrappings, contrasted at this point of the analysis with a body that had broken.)

She goes on to describe other medical studies being done:

M: I had a hysterosalpingogram. Raúl accompanied me yesterday. But I have no companionship from him. He sees many things about me in which I fail him. I avoided arguments ... We have so many clashes that it frightens me. A baby who's going to be in the midst of insults.

In another moment of the session:

M: We are going to have more courage to live for the child.

I showed her that she is the one who needs to have more encouragement to live. With so many clashes, she feels very alone.

She keeps talking about the arguments with Raúl, his jealousy, that "he's jealous" with a girlfriend she has as well:

M: He doesn't want Monica to derail me. He doesn't accept me failing.

Raúl functions as a violent father who "puts his daughter back on track," showing her only one possible path.

Sessions continued and also the studies continue. The diagnosis was reconfirmed: no organic causes account for the infertility. She continued searching for work, and the arguments with Raúl went on.

The question we discussed was why she was letting him do it. What was really going on for her to put herself in that position? She could not defend herself either from Raúl's criticism or his beatings. At this stage of the analysis, she began to be less anxious and more depressed.

M: I feel alone ... nobody comes home. With Raúl's family we don't get together. I also don't see my brother (starts to weep) ... after my mom passed away I didn't see him anymore ... I was sad last week, because it was his birthday ...

She is very sad that since her brother got married, her sister-in-law has "separated them." They have a daughter she loves very much and cannot see her because of the arguments with her sister-in-law.

Her relationship with her brother and her violent link with Raúl became a topic of analysis at that time. She had moments of anxiety, as well as sleepless nights. She insisted on the idea of something to calm her down. She needed something concrete to heal her and felt that words were not enough to support her.

During a session, while she was speaking about her conflicts with her family and her blood relations, something new emerged: she remembered uncles who lived in Cordoba and things she expected to inherit that she didn't know how to deal with.

M: I met my uncle when I was 13. He promised he would come to my fifteenth birthday, he couldn't come …
A: We are back in your adolescence …
M: They are both mom's brothers. In Cordoba, there is also Dad's family. This uncle passed away when I was 21 years old.

When I heard this story, I realised that I saw María as someone alone in the world and that much of the mourning for her mother's death was also related to her orphanhood. She no longer had either of her parents. Thus, listening to the stories of her uncles and closest relatives in her affections, the countertransference experience was that she was starting to have other links in her mind; the things to inherit that she does not know how to face are connected to the passing of time and generational change. María was positioned in a standstill time.

We worked on her feelings of being an orphan, of feeling like a frightened child faced with the world, and not knowing what to do. In this period of the analysis, she talked little about Raúl in the sessions and was more reflective.

At the beginning of a session in the seventh month of analysis, she said:

M: Today I feel a bit calmer. I told him I decided to leave my job. I want to work as a dressmaker at home until I can get something else … I also want to go and visit my relatives in the provinces. Raúl doesn't want me to go …

At the next session, as soon as she arrived, she told me she was pregnant. This was unexpected for her. She was planning her journey to Cordoba to visit her family.

She was ambivalent, not as happy as she had hoped, about the news of the pregnancy, and at the same time afraid of losing it. She said Raúl was very happy.

In the countertransference, I was surprised, though it was something out of place. This was an important moment in her analysis when she was starting to organise her "journey to the interior": a journey that involved her history and subjectivity.

In the following session:

M: The pregnancy continues. I don't know. At night I wake up scared … It caught me unprepared … I have a feeling of hate that I don't know where it comes from … Raúl is more loving but I'm not, I'm surly, and he gets nervous.

We followed this idea of a pregnancy that "caught her unprepared," a "hatred" she doesn't know where it comes from, the impossibility of putting all the feelings and sensations that she was having into words.

What do I think of this situation? Is this pregnancy an accomplishment or a surrender? Is it the resolution of the sterility for which she came to analysis or a new symptom? It was very difficult to think about, but the truth is that the body had spoken again. In the beginning, it spoke from the "mouth of the stomach" and now from motherhood.

For the first few months of the pregnancy, she referred to feeling bad, with a lot of nausea.

M: I've already been three and a half months. Pregnancy is good for me, the rest is bad for me. I sometimes have ankle pain … Ah! I quit smoking. My nerves get the better of me on the other hand!

María's story had no reference to a child; she spoke of the pregnancy. I felt that there was something closer to survival: if it was going to be carried to term, and how it was going to be held and supported.

At the beginning of the fifth month of the pregnancy:

M: It was mom's birthday. I missed her a lot. Sometimes I get very nervous … I miss her a lot, it makes me feel bad … Raúl scares me, he is loving, and touches my belly … It scares me that something will happen to me.

She is more vulnerable with the pregnancy and the changes that are taking place. She doesn't trust Raúl because of everything she has experienced. She doesn't believe in herself to continue living and not surviving. Her mother's death left her in a place of suffering, of pain, and of living at a loss.

M: I can't react to do anything good. I'd like to shout out loud and nobody will hear me! … He says to me: I don't know what to do with you. You no longer pay attention to me.

María was lost, this idea of the visceral shout that is still inside her. As a result of a history of abandonment, she doesn't know what to do with her broken parts.

Her last months of pregnancy were marked by a high level of anxiety and anguish. It began with the phantasy that labour would come early. She recalls that her brother's birth came early; he was born premature. The phantasies of an anticipated birth arose as a scenario of the repetition of her mother's destiny.

María delivered a boy, but he had a birth complication: At birth, her baby's arm was twisted and she had to take him to rehabilitation for several months.

We had various encounters, but we had a closure because her schedule with the baby and his rehabilitation did not allow it.

Before he turned 10 months old, she came back to visit me and show me her child. She was experiencing many financial difficulties but told me that she was better with Raúl, who took care of her child a lot.

Even though the material came from a question about enigmatic sterility, the resolution through the pregnancy presented several questions.

María arrived at the office with grief: her mother's death, a symptom: sterility, and speaking through "the mouth of the stomach." Shortly after she got there, I met another María, battered, with broken bones and a perforated ear.

María was well arranged externally but had broken parts inside. This is the patient I started to listen to. The analysis was based on showing her how she participated in what was happening to her, since she gave the impression that she wasn't in the scene, that everything was "happening" to her.

I felt the impact of the violence María experienced in my countertransference, and each time I was surprised by what she said. It was the baby who was going to give her the courage to live. Her sterility was because of something in her body: the pain in the mouth of her stomach, something she ate.

With the symptom of sterility and "speaking through the mouth of the stomach," she defended herself from loneliness and violence. Discontinued teenage pregnancies such as María's are incorporated as a natural and uncritical event.

In this context, infertility might be considered not only as a defence, but also as retaliation against Raúl: this movement also makes him sterile.

The body area represents a place where symptoms and distress are processed, resulting in physical transformations such as sterility, pains, and fractures. To calm down, she also looks for the transformation of her body through medicine: some external help.

The analysis led her to connect with her history and sorrow. We may conjecture that pregnancy allowed her to re-create her own mother's fusional link. She also worked through the mourning for her mother's death by becoming a mother herself.

María's pregnancy is not "narcissised" in the classical way, which gives it a certain completeness. Maternity is still in a place of resistance; it doesn't conform to its brightness.

The desire for a child, in this case, was a controversial point, since there was no previous birth: her own birth as a subject. In this case, she assumes the identity of "mother" through her gender to give a new direction to her life, but even so there is discomfort in the link with Raúl, and she begins to be more conscious of this fact.

Beyond this point, I do not know which direction she has taken. Therefore, the solution to an intra-subjective and inter-subjective problem is found through motherhood, as in so many other stories. This reveals to us at the same time how the woman's body is the place where complex problems often develop.

This clinical case of "enigmatic" infertility enables us to understand that the psychoanalytic elements regarding unconscious determinants of reproduction are both singular to each subject and also dependent on the social framework.

In France, infertility is labelled *enigmatic* (Frydman, 1986) when there is no known organic cause for the impossibility of conception.

Complexity in the body-mind relation is also seen in false pregnancy or pseudocyesis. These women present both somatic and hormonal changes similar to pregnancy, yet there is no pregnancy. We may recall that at the dawn of psychoanalysis, patient Ana O. (Freud, 1916–1917) had symptoms of a false pregnancy after Breuer had proposed to interrupt her treatment (Freud, 1985).

A classical study by Benedek et al. (1953) elaborates a classic research on the complex connections between fertility and emotional life. These authors point out that a single insemination produces a pregnancy in 99% of cases in animals, whereas in humans the percentage ranges from 4% to 30%. They observed that women with no ovulation disorders began to present anovulatory cycles once artificial insemination took place. They studied six women who had been referred for artificial insemination due to their husbands' relative infertility. After insemination failed, they were referred to psychotherapy. The effects were controversial since one of them got pregnant but panicked and had a miscarriage and the other five did not get pregnant. We can argue that it is a limited study given that it observed only a few women.

Although it has been a long time since the publication of Marie Langer's *Maternity and Sex* in 1951, many of her disturbing questions linger. Her stories offer the advantage of being divested of the advances in reproductive medicine that surround us today. Her observations are rooted in the Freudian and Kleinian theoretical perspectives. This author argues that the difficulties of women experiencing transitory infertility are determined by a strong fixation to the mother with feelings of guilt and fear of retaliation. There is also persistent ambivalence towards motherhood. She wonders why analyses have not yet been able to explain why the same conflict may lead a woman to infertility, a compulsion to conceive, a pseudocyesis, or an ectopic pregnancy.

An author who has further explored the issue is Deutsch (1973). She pointed out that the same psychic problem may be found in women with infertility and in those who have a large number of children as if it were two sides of the same coin.

There are obviously different views on enigmatic infertility, also known as psychogenic infertility. As psychoanalysts, we can say that all infertility is enigmatic, even when there is an organic cause, since something unknown, a remainder, is always left over.

The lost pregnancy: Miscarriage and abortion

The vicissitudes of miscarriages and induced abortions are problematic issues in reproductive disorders. In this section, I develop some ideas regarding their place in the life of every woman and every man.

In Spanish, there is only one word for induced abortion and miscarriage—*aborto*—whereas in English and in French these two notions are differentiated by the language. In English, the term miscarriage refers to spontaneous abortion and differs from abortion in that the latter is induced. In French, the term *fausse couche* is used for spontaneous abortion and *avortement* for induced abortion. The acronym IVG[21] is employed to describe the voluntary termination of pregnancy.

Psychoanalytic literature has barely dealt with abortion, although it is a topic often encountered in clinical work. We may wonder whether it involves something taboo: the woman who does not desire to be a mother. Julio Aray (1966) published an entire book on the topic.

As a socially established practice, induced abortion has been popular and frequent. Medical techniques have been perfected as a result of advances in knowledge of female anatomy and physiology, and the methods became increasingly less traumatic. Despite the popularity of contraceptive methods, this practice has not declined in our culture and has always been considered private, belonging to the female world.

In the 19th century, it was practised in all social sectors. Abortionists reported at least 10,000 cases in London in 1898. Knibiehler (2001) notes that abortion became a political issue towards the end of the 19th century as life tended to be preserved in the face of wars and armed conflicts. Therefore, the search for a way to limit abortion practices began. In France, abortion is regarded as similar to infanticide by considering the foetus and the embryo as complete human beings. At this time, obstetric care has moved from the home to hospitals. After World War I, birth control placed the issue of abortion on the agenda as birth rates increasingly dropped. The practice of abortion was then punished with severe sanctions; however, the results were not as expected, since abortion did not disappear. Instead, it became a clandestine practice with greater risks to women's health. On the other hand, motherhood began to be legally protected by the inclusion of rights such as six weeks of maternity leave after childbirth (Knibiehler, 2021).

After World War II, the so-called baby boom occurred, while clandestine abortions remained a daily practice. They became a cause of death given the conditions in which they were performed. In France, between three and five hundred deaths were reported every year (Knibiehler, 2021).

The rise of feminism in the 1960s introduced the slogan: "a child if and when I want one," divesting motherhood of its status as being natural and every woman's destiny. The struggle for legal abortion continues to this day.

Between the 1960s and the 1980s, voluntary termination of pregnancy was legalised in Western Europe: 1967 in Great Britain; 1975 in France; and 1984 in Portugal and Spain. In the United States, it became legal in 1973. Although abortion is a complex issue to address from a socio-historical perspective, from a clinical perspective it is observable: its effects are inscribed in each life history, and it acquires varying meanings. What is more, it may have a "subjectivising" or "de-subjectivising" effect.

At the same time, the sexual difference between men and women is involved. Pregnancy can be terminated only in a woman's body. For men, pregnancy is another outside his body since the beginning. The idea that it is the mother who can decide whether or not it will live may leave him at the mercy of her will. Sometimes it is he who prompts the woman to terminate the pregnancy, whereas in other cases he is only a passive bystander.

However, the woman is confronted with her decision. It involves her. It is an event that will be re-signified throughout her life. It is a question usually asked of women in medical consultations on infertility though it is rarely considered in men. It is treated as an exclusively female issue, even if it also concerns men. Dinora Pines (1989) points out that not giving birth to a living child, whether through miscarriage or induced abortion, will always have unique effects on each woman. She adds that it is common to find a sense of loss, prolonged grief, and unresolved mourning many years after the event, according to her own experience. She also observes decreased self-esteem and also hatred towards her female body that did not give birth to live children as their mothers did (Pines, 1989).

When an abortion is followed by difficulties in achieving a pregnancy years later, the experience that did not entail major complications, usually in adolescence, may take on a new dimension on a subjective level.

Julio Aray (1966) also addresses this issue. He points out that abortion always involves a double scar: a psychic one and another on the body. He argues that the status of its mourning is different from other types of mourning, since in the psychoanalytic treatment of men and women it often lasts for prolonged periods, either directly or indirectly. He considers that it involves the loss of the object and also the loss of parts of the body ego and the psychological ego. One induced abortion may be forgotten as a mere vicissitude in a woman's life, whereas in other cases it may be re-signified later in her life when seeking pregnancy.

The following clinical vignette illustrates the complexity of phantasies, ideas, and affects around induced abortion.

An urgent decision

Diego (23) and Emilia (21) requested an urgent interview given that they were pressed for time, as they explained[22]. They had been together for five months and gave Emilia's unexpected pregnancy as the reason for their consultation.

Diego said, "She got pregnant. I have a philosophical stance against abortion. I believe we should have them. I feel ready to have a child, but the ultimate decision lies with the woman (...) I need her to be a mother. I know our conversations don't help much. If we'd decided to continue with the pregnancy, I would tell my dad first. I used to tease him. I used to tell him he had a daughter. I was always being ironic."

Emilia remained silent in the first two interviews, as if absent. The couple decided to terminate the pregnancy and in the following interview Emilia talked about it:

> Emilia said, "It was not as traumatic as I thought it would be. Internally, I felt relieved because I got rid of the problem. If I was relieved, it's because I don't regret it. I was afraid, but now I feel relieved that nothing happened to me."

> Diego said, "I'm concerned about fertility. My relief will arrive when I have a child. She thought about death, about herself. I thought about the future instead."

> Emilia said, "The surgery was on Monday. I had to be alone. That was horrible. The following day I stayed in bed. I said I felt unwell because I was on my period."

The couple discontinued consultations after three interviews following the termination of the pregnancy.

Interviews prior to induced abortion as a reason for consultation are uncommon. The attending analyst noted that during pre-decision interviews, the couple referred to it as the *abortion*. However, once it was performed, they spoke of it in different terms: the procedure or the operation. This was a way of detaching from it and assigning it medical status.

The consultation was also contaminated by an evacuative element starting with the very reason for consultation. Emilia's subsequent relief is also a way to put the topic out of her mind by interrupting the treatment, revealing her impossibility to work through what she had experienced.

This clinical vignette allows us to conclude that induced abortion implies a decision and an act. It involves an active search for a professional to perform it and the money to pay for the expenses. At the time they were doing it, it was a secret since it was illegal. Therefore, everything surrounding the abortion at the time it was performed was inscribed within a traumatic situation. This was expressed by Emilia when she said that "being alone was horrible" and when she talked about her fear of dying. It was her awareness of something dying and the marginality involved in these situations.

Regarding Emilia's relief, Pines (1989) observes that for some women, when pregnancy is confirmed, the foetus is cathected as a baby with physical appearance and even sexual identity. For them, abortion is a painful loss, as would be the loss of a full-term baby. Yet in other cases, the foetus is considered a part of the woman's body they can live without, as if it were a swollen appendix.

Pregnancy may also be an unconscious search for confirmation of a woman's female sexual identity. Following Pines (1989), the search only for pregnancy, but not motherhood, is experienced with relief in these cases, with no feeling of loss in it.

Diego associated the abortion with the decision about himself in relation to his father. He also associated it with his own fatherhood along with threatening phantasies about his future fertility. This reminded me of Rascovsky's (1968) article entitled "Notas clínicas sobre el aborto y su trascendencia en el progenitor masculino" [Clinical notes on abortion and its transcendence in the male genitor] in which he highlights the double movement found in castration associated with abortion. On the one hand, it destroys the genital integration achieved by conception. On the other hand, it objectifies female castration phantasies in terms of emptiness and destruction of the female body, following Klein's ideas. He adds that negation is reinforced by the anaesthetics used in the procedure, and therefore it may remain in the unconscious. He points out that the man shares, consciously or unconsciously, the vicissitudes of abortion with the woman (Rascovsky, 1968). His male castration phantasies are also reactivated with varying intensities. I illustrate with a clinical vignette.

When the memory of an abortion arises

Sophie (33 years old) and Alexander (41 years old) told me in their first interview that they were about to start an assisted fertilisation treatment.

Sophie said, "We went to the doctor's on Wednesday. I got out of there feeling badly … I had memories of the abortion. I began to have nightmares …"

Alexander continued, "The doctor explained a little about the process, the egg aspiration …"

Sophie then said, "Aspiration. This word made me sick Like abortion. It's the same thing but in reverse: instead of removing it, they put it in."

Alexander said, "I told her that since it's her body she should decide alone which doctor is the most reliable."

Sophie said, "I got angry when he told me that!"

The analyst enquired, "What did you think at that moment?"

Sophie said, "Yes, there … (referring to the abortion) my boyfriend abandoned me." "I had to decide by myself. A friend recommended a doctor to me. I wanted nothing to do with the procedure. I only wanted a reliable place."

The secrecy around induced abortion emerges in medical anamnesis as mentioned above. In other cases, the topic is brought up for the first time in analysis. In this clinical vignette, we can see Sophie experiencing assisted fertilisation as a reverse abortion. The whole scene of the abortion performed years ago returned and was assigned new meaning by the word *aspiration* spoken in the doctor's office.

Sophie's discourse is in the first person; she refers only to herself. This takes her back to the abortion. However, Alexander's intervention creates a circuit of two that includes a "we".

Sofia was distressed when Alexander told her that she had to decide on her own, since this evoked the feeling of loneliness she experienced when she had had to decide alone to terminate the pregnancy years before. This loneliness echoes the helplessness she had already experienced. We may hypothesise that the situation of the induced abortion was frozen mourning that reactivated when she was advised to undergo assisted fertilisation in the search for a pregnancy.

It is interesting that a single word—"aspiration"—triggered the traumatic memory in this patient. The representations that evoke the abortion depend on the individual experiences and circumstances at the time it was performed: the way it is inscribed and the value of certain words, places, and images.

It may be accompanied by phantasies of a consciously or unconsciously harmed body, as grieving suspended in time. The search for a child later in life updates this mourning.

Marie Langer (1951) considers that the problem of motherhood in women is related to the girl's pre-oedipal bond with her mother. She also argues that the intensity of the conflict is determined by the girl's love-hate ambivalence towards her mother and the fear of retaliation: the phantasised attacks within her body. In turn, Dinora Pines (1989) argues that pregnancy may be desired and successfully carried. Nevertheless, fear of retaliation from the mother if she gives birth to the incestuous child of the oedipal phase may lead to a psychosomatic resolution of the conflict, such as a miscarriage or the conscious determination to abort the foetus. She holds that the analysis of these early conflicts enables the adult woman to continue her pregnancy.

Pregnancy may also be a psychosomatic solution to a psychic conflict of a different nature. Dolto (1983) asserts that a pregnant woman who does not want the child must be listened to, since this may be her only way to find or regain her dignity. She contends that abortion is a significant event with an unconscious dynamic effect, structuring or de-structuring the symbolic life of the woman and the man responsible for this interrupted pregnancy, whether or not they are consciously aware of it. In this sense, she argues that women must develop a sense of responsibility and deepen their femininity; if not, abortion is experienced as a technical effacement. Regarding abortion law, the author argues that it should be changed so that no woman should have to decide without having first discussed her decision.

Illegality and marginality are significant elements that reinforce and strengthen the feeling of guilt and the disruptive nature of abortions. The disruptive element may be re-signified in the search for a new pregnancy as a silent witness still present and active within the psyche. Hence, it is in the analytical space that we may begin to make sense of these complex situations, often silenced by social pressure and by the prevailing sacralisation of motherhood.

An uncanny dream

This clinical case is about a woman who had two miscarriages at five months of gestation, both at the same time of the year.

Claudia was 28 and had been married to Marcelo for three years. She consulted due to a depressive state as a consequence of those miscarriages. In the previous year around the same time, she had lost her first pregnancy and the symptomatology had been the same: low amniotic fluid and foetal death. She had decided to allow herself some time before trying to get pregnant again and also to have medical consultations so as to clarify what had happened and prevent a new loss.

Around that time, her parents separated. It was distressing for her given that she was very close to her mother, on whom she relied to make decisions. Claudia was very dependent on her mother and had difficulty connecting with her own thoughts and desires.

As a result of the separation, her mother was immersed in her own worries and paid less attention to Claudia, which was experienced as yet another loss together with the two pregnancies. It was probably then that room was made for analysis, since her mother was no longer the provider of meaning and advice for Claudia.

The bond with her father was hostile. She defined him as an emotionally distant person, who had moments of drinking and violence. Claudia and her sister, two years younger, saw him very little.

Her sister, Laura, had not become a support for the patient as she had married when she was very young, had two children, and distanced herself from her family of origin.

Claudia started her analysis due to a state of deep anxiety. She reported sleeping badly from time to time and on some nights she was afraid of sleeping. She linked this fear with other fears: the eruption of painful affects, memories, and traumatic experiences that she tried to keep under control in her wakefulness.

Sudden and traumatic pregnancy losses are re-experienced in a traumatic dream: a new dream scenario. Halfway through the first year of analysis, we were in the midst of her working through the mourning of her lost pregnancies. It was then that Claudia had a dream whose main feature was related to causing an emotional impact, almost dream-like, impregnating her whole day with the experiences awakened and reactivated by the dream.

The dream took place on a night she had had an argument with Marcelo. They had had a medical consultation and had been told to take some medicine because of an infection that had been detected. This was an important finding since it could have been one of the reasons for the loss of her pregnancies. This diagnosis of an infection and the administration of medication opened up a new avenue of hope. It also meant a possible explanation for the sudden ending of her pregnancies.

Claudia felt very ambivalent in the face of this new medical information. She felt, on the one hand, optimistic and enthusiastic given that by finding a possible cause, a new loss could be avoided. But at the same time she was anxious and fearful of opening the way, again, for another pregnancy. This was very much desired, but also very much feared.

Ambivalence emerged as a salient axis, both towards the doctor and the analysis. In the medical field, there were questions regarding whether the next pregnancy would be carried to term; in the transference, whether this analysis was going to be a full-term pregnancy or whether it was going to become a new trauma. I felt there was a standing wall of pain and fear to walk through.

Miscarriages, as traumatic situations, create the experience of an abrupt and unforeseen rupture. This imprint is spread through all her links: everything could be suddenly lost at any time.

The rupture of her parents' marriage was also present because even though they had never had a good relationship, the process of separation involved the loss of her mother's almost exclusive attention.

The night the dream took place she had had an argument with Marcelo before going to bed:

> Claudia said, "I told him that maybe I was getting ahead of myself in being this happy, right? But he replied: 'It won't be easy.'"

"I got angry and wept. After that, Marcelo said something he had never told me before: 'I don't like talking about this subject.'"

Her accounts of the dream:

> Claudia, I' ll tell you about a dream I had because I ended up numb. I was on a stretcher in this position (she showed me the position for gynaecological examination). This was a place where they operated on people without actually doing anything, but they acted as if they were doing something. (She places her hand on her stomach and mimics the action of removing something, and at that moment I associated them with faith healers or miracle cures). "I was covered in blood and with that plastic thing on me. I can't remember the guy's face. After that, he would stand behind a door and watch me. After a while a girl came and said, "This thing he's doing to you is fake."

" The talk didn't happen, but the thing on the stretcher did happen, it did happen. The position on the stretcher did happen, the blood did exist."

In this last sentence her voice changes. When she repeats the word "happen," it approaches the uncanny; her voice changes as if she had entered the traumatic scene without a transition the moment she evoked the dream. After some silence, I asked her if she associated it with something else.

Claudia replied, "I don't know. I was very upset. Because of the stretcher ... I was very impressed. It was the blood that shocked me the most."

Claudia narrated this dream with great anxiety. She also said that she had remained very upset the rest of that day, unable to shake off that anxiety.

The dream took her back to the traumatic scene of the miscarriages. What had distressed her most about it was experiencing a reality she had already gone through, because in the dream she reproduced it, she re-experienced it.

In this case, the dream became a new traumatic factor by means of repetition. It was the emergence of something unexpected and uncanny but in another setting: her sleep. We see that trauma has no memory. It is beyond the pleasure principle and enters by sweeping away the protective barrier.

I recalled the dreams in traumatic neurosis described by Freud in *Beyond the pleasure principle* (1920), in which he discusses war neurosis or traumatic neurosis in his patients. He states that dreams are mere repetitions and failed attempts at re-binding what has been overwhelmed: "the shock" in Claudia's words, the trauma, that was beyond the pleasure principle.

Freud describes two features in traumatic neurosis: the first one revolves around the surprise factor, terror; the second one involves some physical harm that usually counterbalances the neurosis itself. Moreover, he differentiates dreams of desire, anxiety dreams, and dreams of punishment from traumatic dreams caused by accidents or unexpected events. In the latter, the function of the dream as a desire to be fulfilled is affected and its purpose diverges. Freud points out that dreams in traumatic neuroses bring the patient once and again back to the accident or trauma so that they awaken with renewed terror (1920, pp. 12, 13).

In Claudia's narrative, anxiety emerged during her dream because, if the anxiety had taken place before, it would have protected her from the feelings of terror and surprise[23].

We understand that a traumatic situation causes such great intensity of psychic excitation in a short time that the subject cannot get rid of them or work through them in any way. The surprise factor is determinant, since these subjects are not prepared to defend themselves.

Thus, estranged from reality, the dream facilitates access to traumatic content but fails in its purpose (fulfilling desires) and also in its function (being the guardian of sleep). It emerges as a new trauma in the repetition of scenes or trauma.

Anxiety arose in the face of a danger known to Claudia: the experience of the loss of a pregnancy.

In *Psicoanálisis de los sueños* [*Psychoanalysis of dreams*], Garma (1956) argues that traumatic experiences are involved in all dreams, which does not invalidate the theory of fulfilment of desires. He points out that there may be one or more underlying experiences in a dream. A traumatic event may also reactivate a similar traumatic experience that transpired at a different time in one's life.

The author adds that in traumatic neurosis the individuals do not consciously perceive the trauma as a memory, but hallucinate the trauma again via attacks, believing they are actually enduring it again. Garma (1956) points out that "the internal" is perceived as having an "external origin" due to the overly intense cathexes which cause hallucinations in traumatic neuroses.

In this dream, it was the experience of reality and repetition that created the greatest emotional impact. Claudia suffered the traumatic event again in her dream, which she expressed in her first associations after the dream story:

> Claudia said, "The talk didn't happen, but the thing on the stretcher did happen, it did happen. The position on the stretcher did happen, the blood did exist."

What did happen, "the external-real," was now on her "inside," which was the new setting of the trauma. She was telling me: "I was actually there, I had those miscarriages. This is something that once really existed and came back into existence now in the dream, as in a time tunnel that reveals a timeless unconscious."

What also existed was the baby that died inside her and was no longer there; it had also happened the previous year with her other pregnancy.

The effect of the traumatic dream is seen in her being "numbed." I would say she was stunned, overwhelmed by the unfathomable and traumatic reality that the loss of her two pregnancies signified, at the same time of year and with the same features.

The transference aspects of the dream can be seen when Claudia says: "The talk didn't happen." I link this with her ambivalent transference towards the analysis: wanting to talk and at the same time not wanting to talk about the subject. This ambivalence surfaces in her narrative projected onto Marcelo when he told her: "I don't like talking about this subject."

Due to the passage in which Claudia said, "This was a place where they operated on people without actually doing anything, but they acted as if they were removing something," together with my association with faith healers, it dawned on me that Claudia experienced her analysis as if it were "surgery," which was bringing up traumatic memories. It was bringing up a part of her body and feelings she was trying hard not to think about through the dream. Repression fails when anxiety emerges.

What was "fake" about the dream might be understood as hostile transference towards the doctor who did not save her babies' lives: a "fake" doctor; the "fake" babies that could not live and her insides as if they were a "fake" space that could not house her children. Was the analysis "fake" or real?

In the light of the emotional mood of this session, it is the dream that was "fake," that deceived her, and numbed her, left her perplexed and unable to discern between dream and wakefulness, night and day, and past and present.

Differences are not abolished but merely confused and blended. This double space alludes to the uncanny (Freud, 1919), since the object-situation is simultaneously internal and external; it is unknown (repressed) and familiar (too well known); it is absent and present.

The disturbing strangeness is related to the resurgence of the scene, which "did not happen" by means of repression, but "did happen." It is not evoked by memory, but traumatically bursts forth in images-perceptions of her dream. What frightens her is not foreign but familiar.

I was later able to interpret this dream as her re-experience of terror using dream language and as an announcement of her "fear of future collapse" upon attempting a further pregnancy. It actually anticipated a memory that could not be evoked but only hallucinated.

In *Constructions in analysis* (1937), Freud points out that when a state of anxiety makes one foresee that something dreadful will happen, it is simply under the influence of a repressed memory that seeks to come to consciousness but cannot. It is the memory of something dreadful that indeed happened.

In this case, anxiety, the original reaction to the disempowered trauma, reveals subjective destabilisation and the presence of a history that returns as repetition compulsion.

Claudia's dream thus sets up a double scenario: the memory of the traumatic situation and the memory of the traumatic dream. It is a double inscription of the same scene: the unexpected miscarriage.

The traumatic dream is the border between the dream (internal reality) and reality (external reality: trauma). It is also an attempt to bind, to process unbound quantities that have invaded the ego.

What developed in the session was at first her psychic effort to recompose and relocate herself in the present. She felt distressed and scared: the uncanny and the repetition were present. By the end of the session, I appealed to our working through on her dream. I said, "This time, it was a dream."

Notes

1 Varicocele: an enlargement of the veins within the scrotum (M. Perco, personal communication, 2008).

2 IUI: the acronym stands for intrauterine insemination. This is a low complexity assisted reproductive technology technique by which the ovaries are stimulated and then prepared sperm (using swim-up or similar techniques) is inserted in the uterus using a cannula (catheter) (M. Perco, personal communication, 2021).

3 Swim-up: it is a laboratory technique by which sperm is selected and prepared for artificial insemination (M. Perco, personal communication, 2008).

4 I refer back to Chapter 1 (Part I) in the section on male infertility.

5 Spermogram: basic and fundamental test to analyse male fertility. It allows us to estimate the quantity, mobility, and morphology of the sperm. It is also possible to carry out other analyses in order to study further the causes of male infertility (M. Perco, personal communication, 2008).

6 Varicocele: an enlargement of the veins within the scrotum (M. Perco, personal communication, 2008).

7 In this section, I present cases of a heterosexual couple, although it should be noted that relationship consultations include single-parent, same-sex parents, and gender and sexual diversity.

8 Cryptorchidism: a condition in which one or both of the testicles fail to descend. It affects around 3–4% of full-term infants. In most cases, the testicles descend in the following six months. If this doesn't happen, hormone therapy can be used. A surgery in which the testes are made to descend and then fixed to the scrotum is the last option. In the latter case, a late surgery may have a severe impact on sperm production, compromising the male's fertility (M. Perco, personal communication, 2008).

9 Couvade: its name derives from the French word *couver*, meaning to incubate. It refers to customs observed in primitive societies when a couple is expecting a baby. The social function of couvade is to reaffirm the role or legitimacy of the father. It is a ritual in which the man imitates the woman's labour pain, stops attending to his daily responsibilities and physical work, and when the baby is born, he immediately places it on his chest, body to body with his child (B. This, 1982).

10 These concepts are developed in Chapter 2.

11 Temporality frequently observed in sessions on reproductive problems is analysed in Chapter I.

12 Freud, S. (1873-1939) . Letters of Sigmund Freud (pp. 17–22). London: The Hogarth Press.

13 Azoospermia: absence of motile spermatozoa in the semen. Uterine malformations: solid uterus, uterine hypoplasia, bicornuate or septate uterus. If they cannot be treated, surrogacy, among other options, might apply. Premature menopause: menopause is the definite end of a person's menstrual cycle; when this occurs before the age of 40, it is called premature menopause. It implies the absolute impossibility of ovulation and therefore infertility (with the woman's own ovum). It is usually irreversible. It may be due to functional factors (hence its similarity to premature ovarian failure, which may precede early menopause) or to surgical causes (bilateral oophorectomy). Oophorectomy involves the removal of the ovary for various reasons and may be partial or total, unilateral or bilateral (M. Perco, personal communication, 2008).

14 Hysterectomy: surgical removal of the uterus. It may be total or partial (the cervix is left intact in the latter) (M. Perco, personal communication, 2008).

15 This vignette is part of a previously quoted paper by P. Alkolombre and col (2000), "Nada por qué llorar. Duelo, dolor y depresión en la consulta por esterilidad" [Nothing to cry about. Mourning, pain, and depression in consultations regarding sterility] presented at the Congress of the International Association of Psychosomatic Gynaecology and Obstetrics held in Buenos Aires.

16 *Transitory infertility* is a concept coined by Marie Langer (1951).
17 Gynaecological laparoscopy: it is an intra-abdominal endoscopy (introduction of a fibre-optic endoscope) that examines the health of female internal genital organs. This procedure enables diagnosis of different pathologies and, when necessary, surgical correction of malformations, ovarian cysts, endometriosis, uterine myomas, obstruction, or adhesions in the tubes. This technique is also used for gamete intra-fallopian transfer (GIFT), an infertility procedure by which prepared semen and ovum are laparoscopically transferred into the fallopian tubes (M. Perco, personal communication, 2008).
18 Endometriosis: it means that endometrial tissue grows outside the uterus (e.g., ovarian endometrioma, presence of chocolate cysts, and peritoneal endometriosis, among others). This condition produces different symptoms, such as mild to severe pelvic pain, pain during sexual intercourse, and fertility disorders (M. Perco, personal communication, 2008).
19 Intrauterine insemination: this is a low complexity assisted reproductive technique that involves preparing spermatozoa in a lab for introduction into the uterus by means of a catheter or cannula. This treatment is used in cases of cervical factor infertility (absence of sperm or low sperm count in the cervix after sexual intercourse via Sims-Huhner test) and for male factors in which sperm quantity, motility, and morphology are mildly affected. It may be also indicated in cases of idiopathic or unexplained infertility: all known studies to test male and female infertility have been run, but the doctors are unable to establish a diagnosis with an organic cause (M. Perco, personal communication, 2008).
20 In vitro fertilisation: it is a high complexity assisted reproduction technique that was developed to treat fallopian tube disorders (bilateral tubal obstruction) by conceiving an embryo outside the human body. Pregnancy is achieved by using an ovum and semen, thereby creating an embryo that is later transferred into the uterus. This technique was expanded to cases of mild to acute male factor infertility, idiopathic infertility, and failures in the application of less complex techniques (M. Perco, personal communication, 2008).
21 IVG: *Interrupcion Volontaire de Grossesse* [voluntary termination of pregnancy].
22 This clinical vignette belongs to Alkolombre et al. (1999, p. 33), *Aborto provocado, trauma y esterilidad. Una perspectiva psicoanalítica*, in *Primeras Jornadas de.*
23 Freud (1920) establishes a difference between fear, anxiety, and terror. He notes that fear is being afraid of a particular object; anxiety is the expectation in front of a known or unknown danger; and terror occurs when one runs into danger unprepared.

References

Alkolombre, P. (2008). *Deseo de hijo. Pasión de hijo: Esterilidad y Técnicas Reproductivas a la luz del Psicoanálisis* [*Desire for a Child: Passion for Child. Infertility and Reproductive Techniques in the Light of Psychoanalysis*]. Buenos Aires: Letra Viva Editorial.

Alkolombre, P., Dunayevich, S., García Laredo, I., Granero, L., Laduzinsky, E., Scharf, S., & Stivelman, F. (1999). Aborto provocado, trauma y esterilidad: una perspectiva psicoanalítica [Induced abortion, trauma and sterility: a psychoanalytic perspective]. In *Jornadas de infertilidad, adopción y fertilización asistida: un enfoque multi e interdisciplinario*, 33–39.

Aray, J. (1966). *Aborto. Estudio Psicoanalítico*. Buenos Aires: Hormé.

Aulagnier, P. (1979). *Los destinos del placer: alienación, amor, pasión* [*The Destiny of Pleasure: Alienation, Love, Passion*]. Buenos Aires: Paidós (1994).

Aulagnier, P. (1992). 'Qué deseo, de qué hijo?' [What desire? For what child?]. *Revista de Psicoanálisis con Niños y Adolescentes*, *III*, 45–49.

Aulagnier P. (1994). Los Destinos del placer: alienación, amor, pasión: Seminario realizado en el Hospital Sainte Anne [The Destinies of pleasure: alienation, love, passion: Seminar held at the Sainte Anne Hospital], 1977–1978. Paidós.

Benedek, T., Ham, G., Robbins, F, & Rubenstein, B. (1953). Some emotional factors in infertility. *Psychosomatic Medicine*, *XV*(5), 485–499.

Bleichmar, H. (1991). *La depresión: Un estudio Psicoanalítico* [*Depression: A Psychoanalytic Study*]. Buenos Aires: Nueva Visión.

Cain, J. (1994). *Psychanalyse et psychosomatique. Réflexions sur leurs fondements, Revue de Gynécologie, Obstétrique Psychosomatique*, n° 10, Paris.

Deutsch, H. (1973) (1960) *Psicología de la mujer* [*Woman's Psychology*]. Buenos Aires: Losada.

Dolto, F. (1983). *Sexualidad Femenina*. Buenos Aires: Paidós.

Ehrensaft, D. (2018). Family complexes and oedipal circles: Mothers, fathers, babies, donors, and surrogates. In *Psychoanalytic Aspects of Assisted Reproductive Technology* (pp. 19–43). Routledge.

Freud, S. (1914). On narcissism: An introduction. In Ed. J. Strachey, *The Standard Edition of the Complete Psychological Works of Sigmund Freud*, Volume XIV. London: Hogarth Press.

Freud, S. (1916–1917). The development of the libido and the sexual organizations, Lecture XXI. In Ed. J. Strachey, *The Standard Edition of the Complete Psychological Works of Sigmund Freud*, Volume XVI. London: Hogarth Press.

Freud, S. (1917). Mourning and melancholia. In Ed. J. Strachey, *The Standard Edition of the Complete Psychological Works of Sigmund Freud*, Volume XVII. London: Hogarth Press.

Freud, S. (1919). The 'uncanny'. In Ed. J. Strachey, *The Standard Edition of the Complete Psychological Works of Sigmund Freud*, Volume XVIII. London: Hogarth Press.

Freud, S. (1920). Beyond the pleasure principle. On narcissism: An introduction. In Ed. J. Strachey, *The Standard Edition of the Complete Psychological Works of Sigmund Freud*, Volume XVIII. London: Hogarth Press.

Freud, S. (1930). Civilization and its discontents. In Ed. J. Strachey, *The Standard Edition of the Complete Psychological Works of Sigmund Freud*, Volume XXI. London: Hogarth Press.

Freud, S. (1937). Constructions in analysis. In Ed. J. Strachey, *The Standard Edition of the Complete Psychological Works of Sigmund Freud*, Volume XXIII. London: Hogarth Press.

Freud, S. (1961). Letter from Sigmund Freud to Martha Bernays, July 23, 1882. In *Letters of Sigmund Freud 1873-1939* (pp. 17–22). London: The Hogarth Press.

Freud, S. (1873-1939) . *Letters of Sigmund Freud* (pp. 17–22). London: The Hogarth Press.

Frydman, R. (1986). *L'irrésistible désir de naissance* [*The Irresistible Desire for Birth*]. Paris: Presses Universitaires de France.

Garma, A. (1956). Psicoanálisis de los Sueños. Buenos Aires: Paidós.

Green, A. (1980). Passions et destins des passions: Sur les rapports entre folie et psychose [Passions and their fate: Relationship between madness and psychosis]. Nouvelle Revue de Psychanalyse, *XXI*, 5–41.

Hassoun, J. (1998). Por qué se dice la virilidad [Why do they say virility]. In *Actualidad Psicológica*. Buenos Aires. 998. Vol. 23, no. 253 (1998). ISSN: 0325-2590.

Knibielher, Y. (2001). Historia de las madres y de la maternidad en Occidente. In *Historia de las madres y de la maternidad en occidente* (pp. 109–109).

Langer, M. (1951). *Maternidad y sexo* [*Maternity and Sexuality*]. Buenos Aires: Paidos.

Le Breton, D. (1995). *Antropología del cuerpo y modernidad* [*Anthropology of the Body and Modernity*]. Buenos Aires: Nueva Visión.

Martin, E., "La historia de un idilio científico," *in. Orgyn,* Buenos Aires, (1994), N° 3, p. 8.

Nasio, D. (1996). *El libro del dolor y del amor* [*The Book of Pain and Love*]. Buenos Aires: Gedisa.

Pines, D. (1989). Embarazo, aborto espontáneo y aborto: una perspectiva psicoanalítica. [Pregnancy, miscarriage and abortion: a psychoanalytic perspective]. *Revista de Psicoanálisis*, Buenos Aires, 798–809.

Puget, J., & Berenstein, I. (1992). Psicoanálisis de la pareja matrimonial. In *Psicoanálisis de la pareja matrimonial* (pp. 231–231).

Rascovsky, A. (1968). Notas clínicas sobre el aborto y su trascendencia en el progenitor masculino [Clinical notes on abortion and its impact on the male progenitor]. *Revista de psicoanálisis*, *XXV*(3-4), 641–663.

This, B. (1980). El padre: acto de nacimiento [The father: act of birth]. In *El padre: acto de nacimiento* (pp. 272–272).

Chapter 4

Psychoanalysis and Reproductive Techniques

The historical and scientific context

It all began on July 20, 1978 in London when Louise Brown was born. She was the first human being to be conceived through in vitro fertilisation: a landmark in the history of human reproduction. In 1982, Amandine was the first French baby born by this technique and, two years later, the first baby from a frozen embryo was born in Australia. Reproductive techniques were rapidly spreading around the world.

At the same time, they ignited debates about their implementation in different fields such as medicine, psychoanalysis, ethics, and religion, among others. Legislation faced a whole new chapter due to the new filial relationships, kinships, and blood ties, in view of the legal vacuum in this new field of parenthood. One of the most prominent cases was related to surrogacy. In 1987, there was a trial for a case known as Baby M in the United States (Annas, 1988). The Sterns had signed a surrogacy agreement with Mary Beth Whitehead, but once the baby was born, she refused to hand over the baby born from Stern's sperm. The couple went to court, the judge initially ruled in favour of the Sterns since he considered there was a contract that had to be enforced. However, a subsequent appeal recognised Mary Whitehead as the baby's biological mother and granted her the right to visit the child.

That same year, a 48-year-old woman gave birth to the biological children of her daughter and son-in-law in South Africa. She was a surrogate, carrying her daughter's embryos, i.e., her grandchildren. In this case, genealogy was modified, as was the canonical concept of generational differences. As Ehrensaft (2018) notes, the combinatorics in gamete donation and gestational carrier cases involved in many parentalities result in an unprecedented family complex.

Another controversial scenario relates to gestation outside the female body, which belongs to the field of research or science fiction to this day. Atlan (2005) published a book on this topic in which he claims that the next stage will be ectogenesis. Although it continues to be science fiction, it is still a disturbing idea, as depicted in Aldous Huxley's book *Brave New World*.

DOI: 10.4324/9781003296713-7

Héritier (1998) highlights that cloning is the instrumentation of the human body reduced to one thing and that it promotes phantasms of selection, uniformity, and totalitarianism. This author points out that in cloning, the presence of the Other becomes ubiquitous: whereas no identity is possible without otherness, the clone is always the other in relation to the original individual.

Debates in psychoanalysis took place in different forums of discussion. Aulagnier (1992) argues that the implementation of reproductive techniques could mean a return to infantile phantasms of a reality where anything is possible. Therefore, she asserted that they encourage and fuel the old infantile omnipotence that was so difficult to renounce in childhood.

In this regard, Michael Tort (1994) argues that medical technological breakthroughs have shaken our symbolic references by altering identities, kinship, and filiation, as Freud's narcissistic wound did. Tort (1994) explains that human reproduction is underpinned by an unconscious logic of primal representations: infantile sexual theories and their phantasms, oedipal determinism, and narcissism. He also emphasises that psychoanalytic research cannot be restricted to saying that science forecloses the father due to the power apparatus of medicine and biology. He affirms that the implementation of reproductive techniques is a social phenomenon, not just an individual phantasy. Therefore, he thinks that there are two simultaneous realities at play given their collective nature: knowledge and medical technology on the one hand and sexual relationships on the other.

I believe this last argument is essential to understand the scope of *the new order in procreation* from 1978. In the course of time, assisted reproduction as a collective practice gave rise to a new imaginary of the body which is technologically completed (Alkolombre, 2018).

During the 1990s, heated debates focused on the fate of embryos with no parental projects that were accumulated in fertility centres. Not only was this a concern for science, but it also reached the media. The alternatives discussed ranged from destroying the embryos, donating them, or keeping them frozen; this debate continues today.

Another topic of discussion was the pre-implantation genetic diagnosis, a practice similar to embryo selection. In this area, Jacques Testart (1986) raised his voice and asserted his position regarding scientific research on human embryos. He also noted the need for a multidisciplinary approach in the debates regarding the significance of scientific production.

Unprecedented articulations among blood ties, biological filiation, and social filiation raised additional questions. They revolved around effects on subjectivity and especially the question of anonymity regarding gamete donation. It is an issue that concerns the origins of children born through gamete donation whose anonymous heritage would continue to be silenced in future generations.

In psychoanalysis, we reflect upon this *new order in procreation* via practices that have revolutionised the way of becoming a parent. The clinical scenarios that we encounter are concerned with how to be parents through different methods and to have children of different origins.

In the book *Les procréations médicalement assistées: vingt ans après* (Frydman et al., 1998), the authors share their two-decade pioneering experience in the field of assisted reproduction. They state that reproductive techniques signify a revolution similar to the discovery of oral contraception. Throughout the book, they wonder how demands for treatments have recently evolved along with the new relations between biological and social filiation. A strong proposal is brought forward in the book: to maintain a multidisciplinary and pluralistic dialogue in which clinical work should be at the core. As stated by these authors, I consider this project to be a fundamental point in order to be able to continue questioning ourselves critically on the basis of psychoanalytic practice. In this regard, Sylvie Faure-Pragier (1998) considers that each new technological advance impacts at two levels: in reality and within the psyche, where they are re-signified in the *après-coup*.

Parenthood today: What's new?

In this section, I propose to consider the novelties in today's parenthood. To do so, we enter an area in which the correlations between kinship, blood ties, and filiation coexist in exclusion and inclusion. In the area of multiple filiations, we may encounter different combinations both in the donation of gametes and in surrogacy.

Surrogacy began to be requested by women who for different medical reasons were unable to carry the pregnancy to term. Years later, it expanded to men with a project of single fatherhood. We know that today a man can decide to become a father through ovum donation and surrogacy. Initially, some of these men have reached out to the media as in the cases of the singer Ricky Martin as a single father and Elton John together with his husband. Thus, new male scenarios in parenthood were also established (Alkolombre, 2009). It should be noted that in this and other practices we include the complete spectrum of gender identities.

In turn, insemination from a sperm bank is an increasingly growing practice. In my experience, women who are not in a heterosexual relationship decide to become mothers using this technique, although there are other reasons.

So far, we could say that we are facing new parenthood as analysed by Roudinesco (2005) in her book *La familia en desorden* [*The Family in Disorder*]. However, if we travel back to ancient Rome, we find that there was a custom in which a man could temporarily lend his wife to a childless couple in order to become what we now call a surrogate. In other words, she became the woman who carried and delivered a baby for another couple. It was an agreement between men, and women had no say in the subject, as described by Héritier (1992). This Roman practice may now be regarded as a precedent for surrogacy.

Therefore, we can argue that motherhood and fatherhood belong not only to the private sphere, nor are they merely an expression of a desire inasmuch as they simultaneously respond to social needs and their parameters vary from culture to culture. Both the status of male and female roles and sexual and gender diversity are independent of biological sex. Therefore, there is nothing new under the sun.

Nonetheless, something different occurs with the arrival of the children. I would like to ask the initial question again: is anything new about today's parenthood? This led me to think about the new family configurations: assembled, homoparental, and single-parent families, which nowadays coexist with traditional families. But I also reflected on the rupture brought about by the implementation of reproductive techniques. It implies thinking about who will display parental roles as well as how those children will be conceived and brought into this world. It is here that we face unprecedented elements and new ways of conceiving children, something unheard of in history. What used to exist only in myths or science fiction is our reality today. New origins of children pose new questions and enigmas to solve.

Dilemmas about new origins

Different generations live in a culture that is undergoing rapid changes in the field of reproduction. Hence, a new order in sexuality and reproduction is established, new modes of coexistence between genders are enabled, and there are changes in power relations. Until this time, being born meant coming out of the body of a woman who was in turn the child's mother. The reality of genetic testing and the new architecture of human fertility is reflected in clinical work by novel and dilemmatic scenarios related to the origins of children born through assisted reproductive technology.

We all agree that beyond biology, it is parenting that transmits psychic life, and parenting functions are independent of gender. It is nevertheless important to reconsider the place of bodies and desires.

From my point of view, two technological advances represent a break from what was previously known: ovum donation and surrogacy. Gamete donation leads us to differentiate what is one's own body from what belongs to others. It also leads us to consider the inclusion of new categories in parenthood, such as father and genitor or mother and genetrix. Surrogacy, in turn, poses a splitting in motherhood: a pregnant woman who gestates the baby and a woman who desires to become a mother.

In our consulting rooms, it is usual to meet individual patients or couples that are about to undergo or are already undergoing fertility treatments. An issue typically found in cases of parenthood via reproductive techniques is the prospective parents' uncertainty about how to explain their children's origins to them. Hence, preparatory work is essential in each case to enable them to "subjectivise" the experience.

A further element to attend to is the relationship established with technology since it may be at the service of desire for parenthood or at the service of disavowal. The implementation of technology is inextricably linked to the identity of the child to be born, representations in the parents' unconscious, and their projections. These fertility treatment experiences establish new inscriptions rooted in novel articulations between blood ties, filiation, and kinship, as we said.

The analyst's countertransference should be also considered here since it is in the field of immanence: not only does it have an ideology but it also produces it.

I show some clinical vignettes that open questions of a dilemmatic nature concerning the experience of becoming parents via different techniques and having children of different origins.

The doubling out of maternity

When Natalia and Guillermo's foetus was diagnosed with a severe malformation incompatible with life, they decided to terminate their five-month pregnancy. An emergency arose during the caesarean section: a haemorrhage that jeopardised Natalia's life. Therefore, the uterus had to be surgically removed. No sooner did she recover than she inquired about surrogacy and international adoption. In her first consultation, Natalia said, "I will have a child even if they have to open me up from head to toe."

Guillermo added, "She is a bulldozer."

Natalia replied, "I can't wait my whole life, and then it may never happen."

A friend of the couple's, Carolina, offered to carry the pregnancy to term, and they quickly accepted. Natalia said: "I still have my ovaries, that is a sign that shows me where to go next … It could be a new little house for our baby."

The couple hurriedly accepted the offer and started the procedure of surrogacy. Once the pregnancy occurred, the duplication of the bodies manifested itself. Natalia arrived at the session in distress and said, "Today I'm Chucky. I feel like I'm pregnant but I'm not." The figure of *Chucky* emerges in her associations, a doll that seems to be a toy, yet is terrifying. It conveys an experience linked to the phenomenon of the double, something uncanny (Freud, 1919) which comes to light though it was intended to remain hidden. Natalia felt she was pregnant, and yet she was not. In this couple, the resolution of their mourning for the interruption of the pregnancy and all possibility of conceiving a child evokes ominous phantasms of castration. The traumatic origin intertwined with this new parenthood.

An imposed paternity

Pablo was 40 years old, had been separated for 9, and had a pubescent daughter. He attended a session to consult about a difficult decision when his ex-wife wanted to have another child and asked him if he could be the biological father. However, she also made it clear that if he did not accept, she would have the child through a sperm donor.

In his first interview, Pablo said, "As a man, having only one child is too little. I'm not complete, I have more to give as a father, and my daughter needs a sibling. I've been thinking about it carefully, I can't stop thinking."

A few weeks later, he came to a decision: "Finally, I told her 'yes', because if I had refused, that child would be born anyway, and my daughter would have a sibling with no father. I'd rather look after a child of my own than nobody's child," Pablo said. He arrived at the decision from his role as a father, thinking that the child would be a sibling for his daughter. The roles of the genitor and father are at stake here, since his ex-wife equated him to a donor by asking him to be the biological father of the child, i.e., the sperm provider.

Some expressions can be extracted from the session such as "nobody's child" and "a sibling with no father" when referring to a child born via a sperm donor. In this regard, it was Pablo who could be an agent of his own desire in the face of this dilemma posed by his ex-wife and come to a decision.

A being from another planet

Pedro and Karina arranged an appointment in their second month of pregnancy. They had used ovum donation, since Karina had had an early menopause, her menstruation stopping when she was 35. In one of the sessions, there was anxiety in Karina. She feared that something bad would happen and had second thoughts about using a donor. At some point, Pedro said "I imagine you may feel strange with a pregnancy like this one, as if you had an alien. You don't know where it comes from!" The idea of the *alien* becomes strong. It is a child coming from another planet, an *alien* from another unknown "body-planet," from the body of another woman, the donor.

In this session Karina raised a concern regarding the possible "siblings" her child may have and the risk of incest given that her treatment involved a shared donor: the other portion of the ova was donated to another woman.

Karina said, "One wants to know more ... what do I have inside my body?"

In the next session, she shared a dream:

> I was hanging from the outside of a window and my fingers were slipping, I feel like I'm falling into the abyss. At that moment some cousins, who are not my cousins, came and dragged me inside. I told them, Thank you, girls. These cousins are not my genetic cousins, yet we were raised together. They are like cousins, but they are not and in the dream, they didn't let me fall off the cliff.

There were associations regarding the women who helped her, as did the ovum donor in rescuing her from the risk of not becoming a mother. There were also concerns about the origin and genetics of her future child. The central element of this session was the figure of the cousins, who represent a familiar bond of affection. Although they were not genetically cousins, they did share an emotional bond, in the same way the child Karina and Pedro were expecting shared a bond with them, although they were not genetically related. This couple continued their analysis given that they moved from a child perceived as an alien, a being from another planet, to a child seen as the cousin, from a familiar affective bond.

Where do they come from?

Carlos and Marta resorted to both egg and sperm donation after several failed fertility treatments. In their sessions, they barely talked about the donors; they were more concerned with the course of the pregnancy. Around the fifth month of pregnancy, Carlos, who was visibly distressed, told Marta, *And where do the embryos come from? There's a kind of void; what will they be like? What if they're Chinese?*

Carlos' question permeated the session and aimed at the unsaid and unknown about the origins of the expected child: Chinese, a foreigner. It reminds me of Pedro's figure of the alien, Pablo's nobody's child, and Natalia's Chucky. These representations border on everything unknown and unsettling they are experiencing. These elements lead us to rethink origins as a founding place in our clinical work.

It is unprecedented origins that establish a radical difference. Hence, they need to be further worked through. We are aware that origins have fundamental importance for the subject. We wonder about the effects on parenthood and children who are unable to ascertain their biological precedence. There is no unequivocal answer to these questions in our clinical work.

Although there is much to reflect upon in these clinical vignettes, I focus on the effects of what I call (Alkolombre, P. 2017) *the new order in procreation* brought about by reproductive techniques. It is an order in which sexuality and reproduction become radically dissociated. The place of the bodies develops into a central topic in representations and fantasies in relation to facing anonymous external genes, or when their child is being hosted in another woman's body. In this regard, novel origins form a new vector within the subjective and social fields.

Donors becoming genitors emerge, expressed in different representations that reveal an effort of binding in the presence of the unknown. Images and words give "figurability" to something external to the bodies, an area with blurred boundaries between what is one's own and what belongs to others. Becoming parents in a modified way and having children of different origins demands extra, additional psychic work that stems from the new ways of conceiving children. In view of these changes, the analyst's permeability is challenged.

An ultrasound of the mind

The way we psychoanalysts understand our patients' narratives is not a minor issue. Faure-Pragier and Pragier (1987) in turn point out two conceptions of mechanisms involved in infertility, depending on whether it is a symptom with a specific meaning or a non-specific psychosomatic response. Bydlowsky (1998) makes an interesting point related to this topic. According to her experience, it would not be suitable to refer to the psychic causality of infertility since it is a medicine that presents biological dysfunctions in a system of linear causality. Hence, the psychic aspect would be within medical logic. This author argues that we cannot discuss psychic causes in the same way as ovarian or spermatic causes. Instead, she suggests thinking about psychic risk factors in infertility.

The type of bonding between a woman and her childhood mother, a frequent and clinically observable element, appears as one of these risk factors: the mother of tenderness, of devotion, often forgotten or repressed. A further element of analysis within maternal identification is the adolescent's envious feeling of hatred towards her mother's pregnancies. This feeling of envy may be extremely powerful and therefore conceal the original infantile love for the mother. She also presents oedipal reasons: paternal nostalgia allows no man in the woman's generation to measure up to her childhood father. Lastly, she points out that there are unknown factors found in women, which she calls unyielding to in vitro fertilisation. These women undergo many unsuccessful treatments, since infertility protects them from underlying, deeper conflicts.

From my clinical experience, I would add that there are also cases in which an actual tragedy has occurred: women whose mothers died in childbirth or suffered a puerperal psychosis. Assailed by tragedy, these women identify with a mother who has succumbed to motherhood, as in Winnicott's *fear of breakdown* (1991). These women have an unconscious fear of suffering the same catastrophe if they become pregnant. I remember the case of a woman whose father had suddenly passed away when the patient was five months old. At the time of the first interview, the couple had been seeking a pregnancy for three years and had undergone several assisted fertilisation treatments. After some time, she became pregnant, yet she feared something wrong would happen to the baby or her husband throughout her pregnancy. Once the child was born, this fear continued to cause her great suffering and anxiety. The shadow of that childhood tragedy remained present. She remembered that there were no photographs of that period of time given that her mother was in mourning.

Infertility may also be a defence against depression: the transmission of life is interrupted for unconscious fear of a psychic breakdown in case of becoming pregnant. There may be a double risk; in some cases, the medical fertility treatments may fail altogether; there may be a risk of decompensation if pregnancy is achieved.

In relation to these questions, Aulagnier (1992) says that it is impossible to generalise or diagnose a psychopathology *a priori* in those who undergo assisted fertilisation treatments. However, she asserts that the possibility of believing again in the illusion of the power of desire is indeed available.

The theory of recursion posed by Pragier and Faure (1987, as cited in Casanova, 1992) offers another perspective to think about clinical work. These authors argue that waiting for pregnancy produces fear that awakens hostility against the woman's mother and regression to the little girl's envy. However, this persecutory aspect is denied and returns as the infantile feeling of impotence. This movement is inscribed as a reversion in which the effects of infertility, in turn, become its cause so that they work retrospectively on the psychic conflict that created them. The authors describe a recursive model in which the consequences are at the same time producers of the process itself: it is self-produced by a source, temporary infertility, that fuelled its first appearance.

I believe these ideas provide more adequate answers within a clinical practice that is always evolving. The psychic processing resulting from medical diagnosis is rewritten and re-edited in each subject in a singular way. I remember the impact of the results of a spermogram on a patient, since it showed several morphological alterations. He fainted in his house that day, stayed home from work the subsequent days, interrupted his daily life, and stopped seeing his friends. During a session, he associated this experience with his father's death due to prostate cancer. The results of the spermogram regressed him emotionally to prostate cancer and the subsequent death of his father. They were associated with the diagnosis. Death anxiety and castration anxiety converged in a double mourning process. Infertility was equated with the risk of death.

What do I desire? From what child?

The analyst often intervenes in cases in which medicine is considered to have failed. Some patients are referred to a psychoanalyst, although the patient does not know why or for what purpose. In these cases, we do not receive a request for analysis but rather a reverse demand: it is the analyst who has the desire to analyse. However, the consultation becomes a privileged place where patients can talk about what they are experiencing: medical exams, surgeries, and different kinds of tests. In this respect, the initial interviews resemble other medical referrals: the patient is referred, yet has no request for analysis. Narratives about medical tests and transference within the medical field tend to prevail. In these cases, there is greater tolerance of physical pain than of the underlying psychic pain. It is also true that an analytical consultation, framed by a medical consultation, has singular features, as noted by Faure (1985), "Except in the case of misguided patients, in a gynaecological visit, the demand is always elsewhere. It is in neither analyst nor patient but is connected to and identified with the gynaecologist" (Faure, 1985, p. 59). Assigning importance to listening openly to those who consult is a field to explore.

From a psychoanalytic standpoint, we may expand the perspective and wonder about the desire for a child and its varying expressions in assisted fertility treatments. In the 1990s, Monette Vacquin (1989) addressed the topic of assisted reproductive technology in her book *Frankenstein ou les délires de la raison*, in which she examines the phantasms involved in the desire to manufacture a human being without sexual intercourse. She argues that infertility is a pretext, but not the underlying reason for the scientific deployment related to new technologies. The author explores Mary Shelley's *Frankenstein*, a novel that narrates the creation of a man in a laboratory with no intervention of sexuality, thereby creating the myth or phantasm of Frankenstein. In her book, she questions the search for knowledge about origins, since the price to pay for it would involve scientific truth obscuring each subject's truth. Shelley's novel also paves the way for ideas of the "phantasmic" of self-conception and the omnipotence that leads to the monstrous. These are Vaquin's delusions of reason.

In turn, René Kaës (2001) argues that the introduction of a third medical-technical element in procreation radically changes birth and representations of procreation. He considers that the latter is achieved by three parties, thereby showing medical technology as a fertilising parental instance. He wonders about modifications introduced in generational relations and the status of the child. He adds that the effects of these technically assisted births on representations of filiation remain unknown. He also observes that although gaps between generations are necessary for their differentiation, their effects are particularly salient in this case and require some kind of resolution.

The truth is that we will only be able to answer these questions as psychoanalysts at a later stage, based on each particular circumstance. It is impossible to generalise the psychic questions these demands may involve.

From "delusions of reason" to the different paths motivated by the desire for a child, we are undoubtedly facing a shift of the paradigm that was valid until the end of the 20th century regarding ways to access parenthood. Thus, at present, when patients face difficulties to achieve a pregnancy, they find other means to become parents. Therefore, we analysts wonder, along with Piera Aulagnier: which desire and for what child?

Undergoing fertility treatments[1]

If we wondered whether there are differences between natural and assisted fertilisation and we believed they are not the same, how would we think about this? What categories would we use? Can this be explained or is it still ungraspable? Guerin (1986) named his book *The Inconceivable Child* to address both the conceivable/inconceivable regarding reproduction and the possibility of thinking about it. They are usually inaugural experiences, different from the way their parents, grandparents, and all previous generations conceived.

When pregnancy results from genetic material from a person foreign to the couple, we reflect upon how uncanny or idealised this might be. When it comes to deciding on the fate of frozen embryos, what does it mean to know that there are still dormant possibilities of becoming parents? After years of searching, when is it time to consider adoption? What would be the adopted child's role? How would the adoptee be inscribed at an intra-psychic and inter-subjective level? How are those experiences transmitted when exercising parental roles?

We have yet to find appropriate words in the language to describe these new filiations, as if there were not enough words to give shape to the kinships of children born of other origins. Tort (1994) discussed natural and artificial kinships. At the same time, we analysts encounter new categories: the embryo is timeless, fresh, transferable, and cumulative; donated gametes, ova and spermatozoa, could be idealised or persecutory phantasies. We also note that "biological child" is a category already built into the social imaginary. The adopted child must build a filiation that depends on recognition, and therefore, we may argue that they have a double birth. Instead, the category of children born by means of reproductive technology is still under construction. Here, the child is both part of a shared lifetime project of couples as Puger and Berenstein (1992) refer to it and also of individual projects. The search for pregnancy develops into a new organiser of everyday life through medical consultations. The monthly calendar is at present limited to ovulation and menstruation dates.

Cathie Silvestre (1989, as cited in Tubert, 1991) introduces the idea of an intersection of temporalities when pregnancy is delayed. There is the present with repetitions of its cycle and relapses of hopelessness. Then, there is the past of a singular history with its own signifiers in the succession of generations. And finally, there is the future of the child to be born, which represents the projection of a desire for immortality and survival.

When analysing couples, the physical presence of the other in the session determines the emergence of new dimensions of clinical material, which differ from a patient's discourse in individual treatment. This idea can be extended to the way the actual presence of donated genes, of multiple gestation or other combinations, operates in the mind of the parents. These aspects are all associated with the body, its material quality, and its density. This presence may be transmitted in a verbal or preverbal manner, consciously or unconsciously, and may trigger phantasies about the child. In this respect, each child has a preceding history: the prehistory of the child to be born, which marks how the child is expected and what their actual existence later represents in the parents' unconscious and projections.

To what extent do technology-mediated modifications in biological conditions bring about changes in parental roles? Are we contemplating a new façade, or is something novel introduced by new techniques and demands? To paraphrase Freud, what are the psychic consequences of technologies applied to reproduction?

We should reflect upon the scope of this topic from a psychoanalytic standpoint and upon the dimension in which experiences are inscribed in patients. Some elements may refer to the patients' history, their phantasms, oedipal process, identification models, the use of their bodies in conflictive situations, and their role in family dynamics. However, reproductive technology introduces new elements stemming from a shift in the representation of begetting privately.

The issue of assisted fertility comprises both the ethics of science and the ethics of love. It is a field that has not been around long enough to evaluate results. This is the first generation of parents with children born by means of these techniques.

Questions bring effects back to our practice. Patients arrive at our office with new sources of suffering. Couples face the dilemma of using a sperm donor or deciding on adoption; others move forward with the idea of surrogacy. Some couples ask for the donor to be a relative, clinging to the phantasy of not introducing "foreign" blood into the family. We also find the coexistence of a profound marital crisis with unbroken continuity in fertility treatments that promise a saviour child to keep them together. Other couples undergo traumatic mourning, displaced by mourning for the child who does not arrive. We also listen to insemination requests by single women who exclude men and develop the phantasy of parthenogenesis; we also listen to enigmatic infertility in women who unconsciously reject motherhood.

Similarly, men diagnosed with infertility may have paranoid fantasies when faced with castration anxiety. In some cases, donation of spermatozoa works as resolution in the eyes of society. It coexists with conscious acceptance of the donation as a defence mechanism to deny infertility.

This clinical work has specific features that may present challenges. The very roots of humankind and human identity were affected by assisted reproductive technology 30 years ago. Hence, although it is no longer possible for us to think of a baby born from a rib, some issues about fertilisation treatments involve elements that are difficult to consider as representations.

The analysis of some new elements introduced by reproductive technology enables us to deepen the understanding of its effects:

- Disjunction between sexuality and reproduction
- Desire for a child/desire for pregnancy with oedipal or narcissistic predominance
- Breach in the time-space axis: date of conception versus date of embryo transfer

- Breach of the generational gap and family links
- Role of the donor: third party, excluded from the couple and their projections of the child
- Phantasies of parthenogenesis
- Denial of gender differences
- The feeling that the child is an exceptional being

It is difficult to describe the best conditions for the subjectivation of these experiences and the arrival of these children into the world. Aulagnier (1992) argued that it is impossible to generalise or make any *a priori* psychopathological diagnosis of couples who require assisted fertilisation treatments. However, she states that what is certain is the possibility of believing again in the omnipotence of the desire that was so difficult to abandon in childhood.

Similarly, we analysts are challenged to unveil the unconscious wagers in these consultations and to question the effects of these new practices.

An individual treatment

I will discuss the dream of a patient I treated a few years ago. It is the case of a 40-year-old woman who desired to have a second child. My patient had a successful professional career; she had a daughter, Alejandra, who was 11 years old.

Before consulting, she had already undergone two unsuccessful fertility treatments. In our session, she recalled that the night before, her husband had woken her because she was screaming in her sleep; she was extremely distressed and upset. At that time, she was working through the possibility of not having a second child. She did not know whether to attempt a new fertility treatment or not; she was ambivalent.

Her narrative of the dream:

> … I was with my husband and so was Alejandra. Suddenly, Alejandra turned into a little box, a little cardboard box …

When asked about possible associations, she could not think of any. I asked her if this could be related to what we had been working on concerning motherhood. She replied that it might be and remained silent.

At that moment, I considered this might be the patient's phantasy to re-experience Alejandra's pregnancy so that she would be a small child again inside her womb-box, still unborn, fading from her perception. This way, she would re-create a successful pregnancy in a hallucinatory fashion. I shared this interpretation with her.

She told me that she had been feeling deep anxiety. She feared that something bad might happen to her daughter. She had suffered severe anxiety crises due to her father's death when she was a baby. I showed her the relation between the birth of Alejandra and her father's death.

When I asked her whether there was anything else she associated with the dream, she answered that it was a little grey box. She considered it and said, "… grey, made of cardboard, like those little boxes that contain eggs, Easter eggs."

I was struck by the thought of the embryos not born in her previous attempts at assisted fertilisation, which could have been other Alejandras, other children. Yet I doubted whether this would make any sense. I admit I find this association strange; however, it was the issue I had associated it with. It was a phantasy about the embryos, and my interest thus shifted to the laboratory: the "little boxes" in which the eggs, the embryos, were kept. I found it hard to think about it and even harder to articulate it. Nevertheless, I decided to move forward along this line of thought. The little box containing eggs could represent the embryos she had had inside her body but did not manage to implant. I presented this idea as a question.

The patient began to cry. She said she was extremely sad and anguished. She told me she wanted to decide whether to try a new treatment. She felt that given her age she could not wait any longer. The little box with eggs also represented her biological clock, the passing of time connected to fertility.

It was a dream that made a considerable countertransference impact. Its analysis and implications were hugely important to me.

Notes on the ICSI

The acronym ICSI[2] stands for intracytoplasmic sperm injection. It is used in cases of men who have altered sperm parameters. It meant a possible solution to the unthinkable: a single spermatozoon is needed to fertilise an ovum.

Initially, two schools of thought in the scientific field coexisted: the first one trusted the scientific process regarding the technique. The other one expressed some reservations and concerns about the potential transmission of genetic abnormalities to the children. The truth is that it has a function of reparation for many men faced with infertility.

The arrival of ICSI as an assisted fertility technique marked a revolutionary shift because it addressed medical assistance directly to men for the first time. Its implementation grew exponentially: a single treatment was administered in France in 1991, and by 1996, 12,000 treatments had been performed. These figures show a projection of the impact of its implementation.

Research on this subject was conducted in France by Koeppel (1998) at Antoine-Béclère Hospital in Clamart. It was carried out on a population of 23 couples who had undergone ICSI. All couples had been cohabitants for a long time: the average cohabitation was eight and a half years, and all couples were in the middle class. They had all been actively, though unsuccessfully, seeking pregnancy, most of them resorting to artificial inseminations using a donor or classic in vitro fertilisation.

This research shows the impact that the possibility of restoring biological fatherhood has on couples. It concludes that men did not feel like "guinea pigs" but were thankful and anxious to have children who would carry their gene pool. This was the last attempt at biological fatherhood for many of them.

In order to heal narcissistic wounds, a single embryo is enough to restore the fertilising capacity of men. In this respect, research agrees with Jacques Hassoun's argument regarding virility. He states that masculinity is more strongly associated with the capacity of conceiving than with the arrival of children.

Research indicates that once embryos are formed, the tension and anxiety focused on the man shifts to the woman. Women are full of expectations of being able to become pregnant and carry the reproductive process to term. When this process cannot be achieved, it is the woman who feels responsible, and she therefore shifts from being the "accuser" to the "accused," as pointed out in the research. This emotional shift within the couple is characteristic of ICSI. Research indicates that the levels of anxiety and concern are not the same in patients who have definitive infertility azoospermia (absence of spermatozoa) as in patients whose infertility is temporary.

So far, we may argue that questions raised in regard to the implementation of reproductive technologies return to the effects of the practice. These patients arrive at the analyst's office with novel reasons for consulting. In some cases, the couple's genetic material is used, whereas in others, the genetic material is provided by a third party, which leads us to the issue of gamete donation.

Gamete donation

At present, gametes, ova and spermatozoa, are interchangeable goods combined and substituted in various ways via assisted reproductive technology. Gamete donation is not a medical treatment per se, but rather the process of substituting a missing gamete, an ovum or a spermatozoon, for one donated.

Donation, another's "gift," enables access to parenthood. In this case, filiation and fertilisation take separate paths. Authors Delaisi de Parseval and Janaud (1983) carried out research on the impossible children in their book, *The Child at Any Price*, after many years of working in the field of insemination using a donor. They wonder about limits: whether there is a right to have a child just as there is a right to work. These authors hold that boundaries in the scientific field have been broken down. However, some barriers standing in the social body are in the process of being resolved. In this respect, they argue that society still lacks referents for these new affiliations.

Initially, gamete donation might or might not be anonymous, casting doubt on secrecy, filiation, sexuality, and identity. The desire to donate ovum or spermatozoa to a relative may be understood as a desire to perpetuate filiation and continue the family lineage, thereby preserving blood ties. In these cases, it is understood that secrecy about the origins cannot be maintained, since it could provoke diverse and varied phantasms in children, in parents' identification projects, and in the third party relative involved in donation. Anonymity in these cases enables the perpetuation of family secrets and a new secret: the couple's infertility.

Reviewing history, France passed its first bioethics law regarding medical assistance in assisted reproductive technologies in 1994, when anonymity in gamete donation—ova and spermatozoa—became mandatory. It also established that it should be free of charge and voluntary (Frydman et al., 1998). The law states that anonymity could be waived in cases in which there is a serious genetic disease. In French law, which authorises the distribution of human body products such as blood and organs, gamete donation is performed in the same manner as any other human body product: it is anonymous and free of charge. The embryo is placed under the same category or status as an organ, as stated by Vacquin (1999). The law also allows the adoption of embryos. According to the author, the thorniest issue is the fate of thousands of embryos in fertility centres for which there is no project of parenthood.

There are many questions on this topic: what if the couple separates or if one of them passes away? What should be done with those embryos? What are the psychic consequences of knowing that frozen embryos still exist when the desire for a child is no longer present, they no longer want to have children, or there was simply a change in their life project?

Egg donation

Egg donation, unlike sperm donation, is a modern technique whose first reported case was in 1983 (Saranti, 1998). In France, it was legalised in 1994 after lengthy ethical and legal debates. It is utilised when, for different reasons, women cannot use their ovaries and oocytes to have a child. One of these problems is early menopause, which occurs before the age of 40, primary amenorrhea or absence of menstruation, and menopause as a consequence of surgical interventions in which the ovaries are removed. These are all cases of young women that can turn to adoption or egg donation.

In this scenario, there have been highly publicised cases of aged women who have had late pregnancies. An Italian doctor, Antinori,[3] became famous after assisting in the pregnancy of an aged woman who was closer to menopause than to fertility.

Ovum donation leads us to think about issues involving the recipient woman, the child to be born, and the female donor. In France, the law established that the woman donor must be under 35 years of age, must already have at least one child, and should not be under pressure. For his part, Testart (1986) considers it unadvisable to create ova banks[4] as an equivalent to sperm banks.

In his book, *L'irrésistible désir de naissance*, Frydman (1986b) includes different types of egg donors:

- The donor relative: it is often the sister, another family member, or a friend willing to undergo a surgical intervention for ova extraction. The donation may be direct: the oocytes are received by a person the donor knows. If it is indirect, the oocytes are destined for an unknown woman; the patient receives other oocytes from the bank.
- The passionate donor: they donate voluntarily, altruism being their only motivation.
- The occasional donor: this occurs in cases of scheduled surgical interventions for medical reasons or when tubal ligation is requested.
- The additional donor: the patient under assisted fertility treatment accepts to donate the ova that will not be used. This practice is mandatory in some countries such as Italy and England.
- The paid donor: although this practice is legal in some countries,[5] it is illegal in France.

Donation is carried out by means of hormone stimulation of the donor woman; oocytes are later extracted via a surgical procedure. Spermatozoa are collected by masturbation, which requires no medical procedure. Egg donation entails other techniques and processes involving the body of the donating woman.

Testart (1986) argues, however, that oocyte donation is equivalent to sperm donation. He notes that ova donation is far from the sexual sphere in contrast to sperm donation which does have sexual connotations. As analysts, we understand that this distance is only geographical since both gametes involve each subject's sexuality, whose meaning is unique.

Whether anonymous or not, in cases of gamete donation the transmission of psychic life goes beyond biology, and secrets cross all barriers of transmission from subconscious to subconscious. Muriel Flis-Trèves (1998) describes this transmission as "the choice of knowledge." Until 1994, anonymity was optional in France so that children could have access to their origin in case anonymity was not chosen. Nowadays the law establishes both anonymity and the cost-free status of donation.

The first publication of a pregnancy achieved through egg donation was in 1983; as egg donation increased, research on donor women began. Research was done at the Antoine-Béclère Hospital in Paris by Blanchet et al. (1998), whose sample was women who donated their eggs anonymously, as required by French law. They observed that from the point of view of the donor, the donated oocyte was represented in various manners. One of the groups (50%) "imaginarised" it as a potential life and the meaning assigned was mainly that another woman would be able to become a mother. Another group (25%) assimilated the process to blood donation, thereby trivialising the matter, or from the perspective of organ donation or as an oocyte that is lost every month with the menstrual cycle. The last group (25%) "imaginarised" it as a potential child, as the donation of a child. These women experienced the desire or the fear of meeting that child as an adult.

In this research, the authors argue that the main motivation of the donors was the experience of motherhood: granting another woman access to motherhood. In this population, there were no prior spontaneous or induced abortions or deaths of children that could explain the donation as an act of reparation. They mention that a second reason was identification with the recipient. In this respect, the act of aiding another woman offered them a valued image of themselves. The oocyte became a precious gift and the donation was experienced as a humanitarian act.

The authors mention that conversations with woman donors on the subject of egg donation led to concerns and contradictions that should be explored. Woman donors indirectly re-experienced motherhood. For recipient women, the anonymity imposed by law was a relief since they did not have to decide whether they should reveal the donor's identity. They already felt deeply indebted to the donor.

In this research, egg donation is seen as an act of solidarity of one woman with another, an aspect also observed by Frydman (1986b) in her book. Donation acquires a human dimension with a more transcendent quality.

From the point of view of the children, most of the women believed they should know about their origins. Moreover, research shows that women who received egg donation often do not want to reveal the origin to the child since they fear the child might look for their biological genitor and reject them as their "mother of desire." Researchers also found a phantasm relationship through identification with the recipient, especially in cases in which pregnancy was not successful after embryo transfer.

We may reflect on the importance of psychoanalytic research in this field and of all clinical considerations that would allow us to expand our knowledge concerning egg donation, a practice established in our culture.

Egg donation by a relative

I once treated a woman who had undergone several unsuccessful assisted fertility treatments (IVF). She decided to consult me after her doctor had suggested ovum donation due to her age and limited prospects of reproduction. Her sister, who was married and had three small children, offered herself as a donor when she learnt about this situation.

It was then that she arranged for the consultation. She was deeply shocked. Her possibility of becoming a mother had implications in her relationship with sister: she was her younger sister, with whom she had competed for her mother's love. She had not yet considered adoption.

Her position in relation to fraternal rivalry made her feel that having a child via adoption would leave her at a disadvantage with respect to her sister and her mother. However, agreeing to her sister's offer of egg donation placed her in a difficult position as well. Her case involved a "relational donor," as described by Frydman (1986a).

This issue marked the beginning of her analysis. Facing the possibility of not having children of her own was extremely difficult and painful for the patient since she could not renounce the image of herself having a child of "her own blood." Throughout the analytical process, a conflict between the sisters emerged. Comparisons drawn by their parents enhanced their jealousy. Her family imposed subtle pressure on her through mandates that did not allow her to think freely about her future. She could begin to pace herself in the race for the impossible child. Finally, the couple decided on an anonymous egg donation.

Sperm donation

Unlike egg donation, sperm donation is not a modern practice, given that it has existed since the 19th century. It requires neither surgical intervention nor hormone stimulation but is instead collected by the act of masturbation.

It has long existed as a rudimentary practice, as stated by Monette Vacquin. However, only in 1973, when sperm could be frozen, were sperm banks created in France, called CECOS (Centres for the study and preservation of sperm). This possibility is immersed in a historical context: decriminalisation of abortion together with the possibility of donating sperm at the service of life.

The first inseminations date back two centuries. Their failures did not prevent the church from prohibiting them, since insemination required masturbation.[6] It was sinful to separate sexual intercourse from reproduction.

A publication in 1909 describes a procedure carried out 25 years previously (in 1884), thereby referring to the first inseminations using donated sperm (Frydman, 1986b). The aim was to attend to male infertility. There is a shift from paternal insemination to insemination using a donor's sperm. Thus, a gene pool foreign to the couple is introduced, an action previously considered to be adulterous.

After World War II, sperm donation expanded although sperm was still not frozen. These practices were developed rather clandestinely and in the absence of stringent measures.

It was only after the 1950s that there was a breakthrough: the discovery that freezing the sperm does not alter its fertilising capacity. The first sperm banks were created in France where they acquired legal status in male fertility treatments. They were set up in public hospitals and rules for implementation were formulated.

Around 10,000 children were born through sperm donation until 1986, and 4,000 men were able to preserve their genetic material before undergoing sterilisation for different reasons (Frydman et al., 1998). Initially, donors were single students and were paid. Sperm banks gradually became regulated and, as in egg donation, they had to meet some requirements: cost-free status; anonymity, though questionable from the child's point of view; and the rule that the donor must already be a father and have his wife's consent.

Sperm donation by a relative

Claudia and Fernando were born into highly religious families, and all their siblings had children. After two years of marriage, during which they sought a pregnancy, they had their first medical consultation. Claudia saw her gynaecologist who carried out routine examinations and referred her to a specialist in reproduction. In the process, Fernando was diagnosed with permanent infertility, i.e., his body did not produce spermatozoa. Consequently, the couple was struck by a major crisis. They understood they were facing a dilemma: either they followed the path towards adoption or they considered utilising a sperm donor. Embryo donation did not come up as an alternative.

This crossroads encouraged them to ask for couple therapy. In therapy, questions develop: they reject the path to adoption given that "science" offered the possibility of having children biologically. They factored in possibilities and concluded that if they resorted to sperm donation, their child would be 50% theirs and 50% someone else's. The statistical way they think about their child is odd.

In the course of sessions, Fernando reveals that he had asked his elder brother to be the donor without telling Claudia about it. He reasoned that the foreign element would be reduced this way. The gene pool would stay within the family and the child would have only family genes. Fernando's request triggered a crisis since Claudia's opinion, or desire, was not considered. Finally, his brother rejected the request.

Analytical work led this couple to opt for anonymous sperm donation. They agreed to keep it secret not only from their family but also from the child: a pact of silence.

Donor "sister"

One of many cases linked to gamete donation is that of two friends who discovered they were "donor sisters" (Alkolombre, 2013). They met through social networks while looking for a roommate at university. Along the way, they became friends, and after a while they discovered that they shared the same sperm donor. The novelty here is related to their shared origins. Although they did not know the identity of the anonymous donor, they were able to compare the information in the sperm bank through the donor's number, which revealed their genetic origin.

As in this case, the implementation of reproductive techniques gives rise to new perspectives on the constitution of subjectivity in the face of fraternal ties. There is a split in transmission: one is biological and the other psychic. In the case of these donor siblings, they share a common genetic load on the part of the male genitor. Although we can know that the caregivers exert the parental functions of transmission of filiation, we cannot forget that the absent genitor also occupies a place in parental projections and is part of the subject's prehistory.

"*Donor sister*" can be considered a new category in parenthood, since it exceeds existing denominations, such as brother or sister, or half-sibling when sharing one of the parents. Much research remains to be done. We know that the origin is foundational for each person and is a question that does not have an unequivocal answer.

Surrogate motherhood

The term surrogate motherhood was coined in 1981 by Noel Keane, a lawyer from Michigan. He was the first to consider that women could bear children at the request of couples who were unable to have children due to the absence of the uterus or uterine malformation. In the Warnock report, surrogacy was defined as a practice through which a woman gestates or carries a child in her womb for another woman, agreeing to hand the baby over to the biological mother when it is born.[7]

Therefore, the mother of that child is the one who feels the desire to have children, the mother of desire, and the other woman is the one who carries the child inside her body. Hence, motherhood is twofold: by means of the body of the gestating woman and by means of the desire for a child placed inside another woman.

Therefore, we might speak of "gestational surrogacy" as the maternal function goes beyond the body. This is how the new scenarios developed by the implementation of reproductive technology force us to review traditional concepts of family, mother, father, and child. In cases of surrogacy, new affiliations and kinships are even more striking.

A child gestated in the womb of a woman who will not be their mother can have a different biological kinship, which will depend on the combinations involved. The child may be the biological child of the couple, developed from the couple's genes, and have a surrogate only in the gestational period. Ovum donation may also have a part: the egg may come from the gestating woman or from a third donor. That child will have only one tie of genetic kinship: it will be its father's biological child since the ovum has been donated. Another combination is presented when sperm donation is implemented together with surrogacy. Genetic kinship will be established only with the "mother" of desire, who is also the "biological" mother. The connection with the paternal genes will remain unknown since the child was conceived via a sperm bank. Lastly, a more complex mosaic results when pregnancy is achieved by means of surrogacy, donated eggs, and sperm. The child has no genetic kinship with its parents, nor filiation with the nesting process.

Gena Corea (1986) argues in her book *The Mother Machine* that the surrogate has been considered a mere recipient, an incubator, and an object. She is paid in order to perform the biological role of gestating while leaving aside the feelings and attachments of the gestating woman. She receives money in exchange for filling the gestating role, which thereby transforms a biological state into a financial opportunity for some women. In his article *Surrogacy: a psychological issue*, Edelmann (2004) points out that while surrogacy arrangements have increased in recent years, it nevertheless remains a controversial practice. In his work, he reviews the research on the subject and highlights: the psychological stress involved in this practice, attitudes, the reasons for resorting to surrogacy, the cession of the child by the surrogate woman, the child's development, and the question of the transmission of the child's origin.

Another issue discussed is the attachment of the surrogate to the child during pregnancy. Although there is little research on this topic, it appears that surrogates express little concern about separation from the newborn.

Many women who utilise this service experience the desire to become mothers but are unwilling to endure the temporary or permanent physical transformations caused by gestation (Cano, 2001).

Conversely, there are those who are willing to lend their uterus. Some do it mainly for economic reasons, whereas others do so altruistically, similar to organ donation. They may also try to assuage the guilt felt as a consequence of an *abortion*. In some cases, a close relative (mother, sister, sister-in-law) offers to carry the pregnancy to term, thereby becoming a surrogate mother, as is the case of a South African woman who carried the children of her daughter and son-in-law in her womb.

From a psychoanalytical standpoint, the questions arise and multiply. Once again, we face the transformations of the female body and the child to be born. There is a new nesting place: the womb as vicarious, another place to gestate, other heartbeats, a different blood flow. What effects will they have on the child, on the phantasms of the parents, and on the gestating woman?

We know that the ego is first and foremost a body ego. We should conduct further research in this new field in order to explore the psychic impact of these new births. They are human beings whose genetic architecture challenges everything we know.

A case of surrogacy

The following case led me to reflect on clinical work, not only its problems but also its ethical implications. It was a case of surrogacy that introduced me to two women: the one who wanted to have a child—the mother of desire—and the surrogate.

Silvia was a 35-year-old woman who arrived at my office requesting confidentiality. She first told me that at the age of 16, she had undergone surgery on her uterus. Initially, Silvia did not explain the circumstances, yet it was possible to infer that it was related to a complex abortion. In the following session, she told me her uterus was removed as a result of an infection due to an induced abortion.

She had been married for a year but had never told her husband about her gynaecological problem. At this stage, the possibility of having children emerged in the couple. She described her husband as a kind person: "The relationship is excellent," Silvia said. She did not want to be untruthful to him, yet she did not know how to tell him about her hysterectomy,[8] although it had happened when she was 16. She said, "I want to have his child."

As for her birth family, she said that she was one of seven siblings and explained that she had always been the closest to her father, which made her siblings jealous. She had a twin sister, who was married and had two children. She said she got along well with her, although there were often quarrels with her other siblings.

I was under the impression that this was an unusual case since she told me she wanted to have children, ignoring the fact that she had no uterus. There was something about secrecy and the impossibility of having children in the atmosphere of this first encounter.

In the second interview, she said she was afraid he would get upset about learning about her problem. Silvia said, "You know when something is perfect?" She argued she would like to have children of their own, and therefore surrogacy would be their only option.

A possible consultation for the couple arose as a question. Silvia said that her husband worked long hours and was interested in psychology. However, we began an individual analytical process. Her story took shape: she had a relationship of conflict and rivalry with her mother while she maintained a strong bond of affection with her father.

Silvia explained that she had been on several spiritual retreats because of shame and guilt over her adolescent abortion. In the first part of the analysis, issues related to motherhood were present. Little by little, she worked through the fear of confronting Juan and the phantasy that he might leave her after learning that she could not have children.

At the beginning of a session, she asked if she could smoke, something she had never requested. She narrated a conversation with Juan in which she could not tell him about her problem. She explained to him that she could not have children after gynaecological surgery at 16, but she did have the ova to become a mother.

At first, Juan was puzzled and angry since she had never mentioned this. At that moment, Silvia became greatly distraught and told him she would leave for a while. A few days later, they got together again and rethought how they would continue. In that session, she remembered the surgery and the words of the doctor who had performed the operation when he told her not to discuss the surgery with anybody. She also recalled that, in her childhood, her overwhelmed mother would tell her, "Do not have children!"

After the surgery, her mother told her to keep it secret and to consider motherhood. She had never considered having children with any other partner, which revealed the efficacy of her mother's prohibition. The emotional and economic stability she had found with her current partner had led her to desire to start a family and have children.

After a time in analysis, she met Estela, a childhood acquaintance who had children. Silvia told her about her situation. Estela was interested in Silvia's problem, and they agreed to opt for surrogacy. She brought the issue to the session and asked me if I could meet this woman before moving forward.

My initial feeling of "unsettling strangeness" returned; also the feeling of the clinical challenge of working with unknown circumstances full of still unanswered questions.

Estela was 40 years old; she was married and had two daughters. The elder was 16 and the younger was 5 years old; she had had both daughters with her current partner. She was born in a town near Silvia's hometown and also came from a large family. Estela was the eldest of eight siblings and helped her mother raise them. Due to her early developed maternal role, many of her siblings called her mum. Her parents separated when she was 15 years old and from then on, her father distanced himself from the family, leaving Estela with her mother and her siblings. She started to work as a housemaid when she was 16 years old. She explains, "I paired up young, moved in with my partner when I was 19 years old, and came to Buenos Aires." Later, she told me she had worked as a caregiver.

When Estela was sitting before me, I wondered what could lead her to accept this proposal. Was it only an economic issue? Were there elements in their story that correlate?

After she told me about her birth family and some details about her history, I asked the obvious question, "Why did you consider the possibility of a new pregnancy and why in this way?" She answered, "I thought it would make her happy. Besides, I'm strong and healthy, I'm still young enough. If I were older, I wouldn't do it ... I talked it over with my husband and my elder daughter. I didn't want to have any more children of my own ... and I would never hand over a child of my own."

Her first words showed that Estela was sure this was a situation she could control and she intellectualised it: "The bond is with my body. I was really moved by her situation." She also talked about her responsibilities, what would happen if the child was born with malformations, and "the medical procedures" she would have to undergo.

Later on, she talked about her mother, who was very hard-working, and about her maternal grandmother, who had worked in the fields until she was very old. She emphasised that all her family had strong moral values. Finally, she said that this agreement with the couple would allow her to pay off the mortgage on her apartment, which was substantial.

To my surprise, Silvia's and Estela's stories intertwined, which allowed me to formulate some hypotheses. Estela, the gestating woman, had been a "second mother" for her own siblings; therefore, being the mother of a child of another mother was familiar to her. Silvia, in turn, was a twin sister. Sharing the space with another woman was something she had experienced since she was born. They both had a strong desire for reparation, and yet it was still motherhood between women. How would she experience being pregnant with a child that was not her own child? How would she relate to the situation? How did she picture it? This was unsaid.

This is a strange situation, unrelated to what we know about.

Soon afterwards, the agreement ended due to quarrels between Estela and her husband. Many questions arose in my mind, as did hypotheses to develop. These cases confront us with novel clinical scenarios.

Notes

1 In this section, even though we consider female infertility within a heterosexual couple as an object of analysis, it can also be thought of within the context of female single parenthood and sexual and gender diversity.

2 ICSI: intracytoplasmic sperm injection. The procedure consists of ovarian stimulation, ova retrieval (through aspiration or puncture), and its fertilisation by injecting a spermatozoon into each ovum (micromanipulation). Then, if embryos are formed (one or more), appropriate means are used to implant them in the uterus (transference) (M. Perco, personal communication, 2008).

3 Una mujer de 59 años da a luz trillizos en un hospital de París. https://www. reuters.com'article'oestp-curiosidades-tr... (May 19, 2022).

4 Oocyte cryopreservation: it is a modern procedure to rapidly freeze oocytes. It basically permits a high percentage of recovery of the ovum's capacity to be fertilised after cryopreservation. It enables ova preservation when the patient must undergo oncological treatments as a reserve in delayed motherhood for different reasons or when a high number of ova are obtained through ovarian stimulation. In high complexity procedures, the remaining ova can be frozen for future use. It could replace the cryopreservation of embryos (M. Perco, personal communication, 2008).

5 This last category is taken from Loukia Saranti (1998).

6 This practice and its punishment by the church are mentioned in the chapter "Historical (In) Fertility." Onanism refers to Onan, who was punished for "spilling his seed."

7   The Warnock report, published in 1984 in the United Kingdom, had a great
    influence on ethical and legal literature regarding assisted fertilisation and
    embryology. It was named for Mary Warnock, Chairperson of the "Commit-
    tee of Inquiry into Human Fertilisation and Embryology" (1982–1984).
8   Hysterectomy: surgical removal of the uterus (M. Perco, personal communi-
    cation, 2008).

References

Aldous Huxley, A. (2007). Brave New World (1932). Reading Fiction, Opening the
    Text, 119.
Alkolombre, P. (2009). Nuevos escenarios masculinos en fertilidad asistida: un vien-
    tre para él [New male scenarios in assisted fertility: A womb for him]. In *El padre,
    clínica, género, posmodernidad* [*The Father, Clinic, Gender, Postmodernity*] (pp.
    153–160).
Alkolombre, P. (2013). Hermanas de donante de esperma [Sisters of a sperm donor].
    https://www.pagina12.com.ar/diario/psicologia/9-240188-2014-02-20.html
Alkolombre, P. (2018). Vicissitudes of the desire to have a child in contempo-
    rary parenthoods: Reproductive techniques and the new origins. In *Changing
    Sexualities and Parental Functions in the Twenty-First Century* (pp. 87–101).
    London: Karnac.
Annas, G. J. (1988). At law: Death without dignity for commercial surrogacy: The case
    of baby M. *The Hastings Center Report*, *18*(2), 21–24.
Atlan, H. (2005). *L'uterus artificiel*. Paris: La librairie du XXI Siècle, Du Seuil.
Aulagnier, P. (1992). 'Qué deseo, de qué hijo?' *Psicoanálisis con niños y adolescentes*,
    3, 45–49.
Blanchet, V., Flis-Trèves, M., & Saranti, L. (1998). Du coté des donneuses [On
    the donor side]. In R. Frydman, M. Flis-Trèves, & B. Koeppel, *Les procréations
    médicalement asistes: vingt ans après* (p. 31). Paris: Odile Jacob.
Bydlowsky, M. (1998). "Filiation féminine et relation avec la mère d'origine," in R.
    Frydman, R., Flis-Trèves, M., & Koeppel, B. (1998). *Les Procréations médicalement
    assistées: vingt ans après* [Medical assisted procreation: twenty years on], Coloquio
    Gipsy III. París: Odile Jacob, pp. 125–138.
Cano, M. E. (2001). "Breve aproximación en torno a la problemática de la maternidad
    subrogada." www.revistapersona.com.ar
Corea, G. (1986). The mother machine: Reproductive technologies from artificial
    insemination to artificial wombs. *MCN: The American Journal of Maternal/Child
    Nursing*, 11(5), 357–363.
Delaisi de Parseval, G., & Janaud, A. (1983). *L'enfant a tout Prix* [*The Child at Any
    Price*]. Essai sur la medicalisation du lien de filiation. Ed. du Seuil, Coll. "Points
    actuels", Paris.
Edelmann, R. J. (2004). Surrogacy: The psychological issues. *Journal of Reproductive
    and Infant Psychology*, *22*(2), 123–136. doi:10.1080/0264683042000205981
Ehrensaft, D. (2018). Family complexes and oedipal circles: Mothers, fathers,
    babies, donors, and surrogates. In *Psychoanalytic Aspects of Assisted Reproductive
    Technology* (pp. 19–43). Routledge.
Faure, S. (1985). La question analytique [The analytic question]. In Psychosomatics
    [*Psychosomatique*]. n°1, p. 59.

Faure-Pragier, S. & Pragier, G. (1987). "Les enjeux d'une recherched sur la sterilité feminine" [The challenges of research on female sterility]. *Revue Française de Psychanalyse, 51*(6), 1543–1567.

Faure-Pragier, S. (1998). "Vingt ans après: du déni a la projection" [Twenty years on: from denial to projection]. In Eds R. Frydman, M Flis Trèves, and B. Koeppel, *Les procréations médicalement assistées: vingt ans après [Medically Assisted Reproduction: Twenty Years on]* (pp. 105–124). Paris: Editions Odile Jacob.

Flis-Trèves, M. (1998). Le choix de savoir: L'anonymat du don d'ovocytes en question. In Eds R. Frydman, M. Flis-Trèves, and B. Koeppel, *Les procréations médicalement assistées: vingt ans après*. Paris: Odile Jacob.

Flis-Trèves (1998). L' anonymat du don d' ovocites en question. in Les procréations médicalement assistées: vingt ans après. *[Medically Assisted Peproduction: Twenty Years on]* (pp. 175–181). Paris: Odile Jacob.

Freud, S. (1919). The 'uncanny'. In Ed. J. Strachey, *The Standard Edition of the Complete Psychological Works of Sigmund Freud*, Volume XVIII. London: Hogarth Press.

Frydman, R. (1986a). La femme sans ombre. Le don d'ovocite in *L' irresistible désir de naissance* (p. 137). Paris: Presses Universitaires de France.

Frydman, R. (1986b). *L'irrésistible désir de naissance*. Paris: Presses Universitaires de France.

Frydman, R., Flis Trèves, M, & Koeppel, B. (1998). *Les procréations médicalement assistées: vingt ans après [Medically Assisted Reproduction: Twenty Years on]*. Paris: Editions Odile Jacob.

Guerin, G. (1986). *L'enfant inconcevable*. Paris: Acropole.

Héritier, F. (1992). Del engendramiento a la filiación [From engendering to filiation]. *Revista de Psicoanálisis con Niños y Adolescentes, 3, 22–31*.

Héritier, F. (1998). "Réalités et fantasmes autour du clonage humain," in Frydman, R.; Flis.

Kaës, R. (2001). "Transmisión entre generaciones: efectos de ruptura y efectos de solidaridad." *Transparencia, El periódico de la Escuela*, Asociación Escuela Argentina de Psicoterapia para Graduados, diciembre/marzo, año 2, N° 3, p. 8.

Koeppel, B. (1998). "L'ICSI et les aspects psychologiques." In Eds R. Frydman, M. Flis-Trèves, and B. Koeppel, *Les Procréations médicalement assistées: vingt ans après: Colloque Gypsy III [Medically Assisted Reproduction: Twenty Years: Colloquium]* Paris: Editions Odile Jacob.

Puger, J., & Berenstein, I. (1992). *Psicoanálisis de la pareja matrimonial*. Buenos Aires: Paidós.

Rodrígue, J. M. M. P., & Massigoge Benegiu, J. M. (1994). La maternidad portadora, subrogada o de encargo en el derecho español [surrogate or surrogate motherhood in Spanish law]. Dykinson.

Roudinesco, E. (2005). *La familia en desorden [The Family in Disorder]*. Buenos Aires: Fondo de Cultura Económica.

Saranti, L. (1998). Dix années de don d' ovocites. In Eds R. Frydman, M. Flis-Trèves, and B. Koeppel, *Les procréations médicalement asistes: vingt ans après*. Paris: Odile Jacob.

Silvestre, C. (1989). "La vie dans ce jardín." Paris: Topique 43, Paris [1989]; cited by Silvia.

Testart, J. (1986). *L' oeuf transparent*. Paris: Flammarion..

The World Medical Association Inc., Document 17.N (1987). Cited in *Ética Médica*, Capítulo VIII, parte 2, Colombia.

Tort, M. (1994). *El deseo frío. Procreación artificial y crisis de las referencias simbólicas* [*Cold Desire: Artificial Procreation and the Crisis of Symbolic References*]. Buenos Aires: Nueva Visión.

Tubert en Mujeres sin sombra (1991). *Maternidad y tecnología* (pág. XV). Madrid: Siglo XXI.

Vacquin, M. (1988). *Frankenstein ou les délires de la raison [Frankestein or the delusions of reason]: essai.* FeniXX.

Vacquin, M. (1989). *Frankenstein ou les délires de la raison* [*Frankenstein or Delusions of Reason*]. Paris: Bourin.

Vacquin, M. (1999). Les lois de Bioéthique. In *Main basse sur les vivants* (p 108). Paris: Fayard.

Winnicott, D. W. (1991). El miedo al derrumbe [The fear of collapse] (1961), In *Exploraciones psicoanalíticas* [*Psychoanalytic Explorations*] I (pp. 111–122).

Part III

Historical (In) Fertility

Chapter 5

First Conceptions

Greece and Rome

Throughout history, people have performed rituals to enhance fertility, as recounted by customs, folklore, and literature. Fertility of the land, of food animals, and the arrival of children were equated in most ancient cultures. Greeks, Romans, Jews, and Christians developed regulatory guidelines for fertility and motherhood, some of which are still preserved, in their societies.

In this respect, we can say that motherhood and fatherhood belong not only to the private sphere; neither are they simply expressions of desire, but rather simultaneously respond to social needs, their parameters varying from culture to culture. In every epoch, the society organises methods of union between men and women, their rules of filiation and kinship. Lévi-Strauss (1979) noted that the family is founded on the relatively lasting and socially approved union of a man, a woman, and their children: a universal phenomenon observable in all societies.

In ancient times, women's bodies played a central role, especially considering the connotation of the uterus in the preservation of offspring. Women were deemed inferior to men because of their lesser size, less developed muscles, less audacious character, and blurred social roles. The Greeks wondered whether this inferiority was due to their reproductive function. The answers also came from Philosophy and Medicine. The Hippocratic Corpus, drawn up in the 6th century and early 5th century BCE, stated that the difference between men and women lay in the woman's uterus (Knibiehler & Fouquet, 1983), an organ considered the source and engine of all health disorders in women.

The oldest documents concerning conception and the female body are two Egyptian papyri dated around 1900 BCE. In them, the origin of all women's problems is attributed to a malposition of the uterus; therefore, several ways to re-position it back to its place are proposed so as to restore health. Different female aches and pains with no visible injury are attributed to the woman's womb and its migrations. It was believed that the uterus moved around in a woman's body and could press and disturb other organs (Tubert, 1991).

DOI: 10.4324/9781003296713-9

According to Hippocratic medicine, health was related to the balance of the four humours that constitute the human body: blood, bile, water, and phlegm. From this point of view, health depended on the proper circulation of these humours. Hippocrates' disciples claimed that all female diseases originated in the uterus, the female organ par excellence, which led to the more abundant fluid exchange in comparison to men: menstruation, vaginal discharge, birth, and milk. The uterus was even considered to be alive, possessed by the desire of conceiving children (Knibiehler, 2001). They claimed that pregnancies were favourable for women since they increased the capacity of the female body to evacuate those fluids. If the womb did not have a good blood supply, women were exposed to different diseases and, in those cases, the remedy was marriage. We see how the utero-centrist perspective reduces women to the functions of the uterus, which is seen as the cause of their distress, heal, or disease. This view is not far from the perspective of female mental illness in Freud's times. Let us remember the demonstrations of Charcot's hysterical patients in the Salpêtrière, in this case associated with sexuality.

Plato, like Hippocrates, claimed that when the uterus did not bear children, it caused irritation in women, took away their breath, obstructed breathing, and produced all kinds of illness. In this view, the impossibility to bear children was part of disease and anguish, and also stripped the woman of a valued place concerning the female identity of the time (Giberti, 1992).

Aristotle developed his ideas about the origins of life by placing the male as the motor principle and the female as the material principle. He said that the foetus is contained within the male, who deposits it inside the female. Concordant with the medical writings of his era, he noted that the womb was the essential organ of women. Strength in female health was reflected by pregnancies, and giving birth was the best proof of a woman's health. By contrast, infertility was considered the absolute evil. Of course since pregnancy and birth ensured the renewal of generations. In the second-century Rome, Galen was the medical authority. He highlighted women's inferiority in opposition to men's perfection, arguing that the role of the uterus is to receive sperm.

As we said, the fertility of the land and living species was the greatest concern of ancient peoples. In Athens, in order to foster more offspring, especially in the 5th and 4th centuries BCE, women were encouraged to enter second marriages (Tubert, 1991). Greek wedding ceremonies invoked Demeter, the goddess personifying the supernatural dimension of motherhood; she represented the cultivated land and the earth, the original nutrient. Rituals for women's fertility, such as the Thesmophoria, were festivals in honour of Demeter celebrated by citizens' wives at the time of autumn sowing.

The androcentric perspective

In all cultures, the objective of marriage was the preservation of the offspring, and infertility was a concern. In ancient civilisations, it was also grounds for divorce and a right. In India, religion prescribed that an infertile woman should be replaced after eight years (De Coulanges, 2020). In Roman culture, the role of the mother became part of the legal order through a series of laws that regulated the family context. The first divorce in history, contained in the Roman Annals, was the case of Carvilio Maximus Ruga (cited in De Coulanges, 2020), who divorced his wife because she could not have children and sacrificed his love for religion given that he had made a sacred marriage vow.

The ancient Roman laws included a specific law that forced young people to marry, hence encouraging early marriages and forbidding celibacy, with the aim of reproduction (Dionysius of Halicarnassus, Cicero, as cited in De Coulanges, 2020). In Sparta, the legislation of Lycurgus assigned women the production of children and imposed severe penalties on men who did not marry. The children of married couples were the only ones allowed to continue traditions, as opposed to extramarital children who were considered bastards. Blood ties alone did not constitute the family, since cult ties were also required (De Coulanges, 2020). Marriage was compulsory. Its aim was neither pleasure nor the union of two persons by love; it was at the service of the perpetuation of the family and with it, religion and laws. Hence, the marital bond could be broken if the woman was infertile. However, if the husband was infertile, a brother or other relative of the husband had to replace him, and the woman had to join that man. The child born from this union was considered the husband's child and continued his tradition of worship.

Sparta required a trial marriage (Tubert, 1991) until the woman's fertility was verified. If it was not confirmed, the marriage was annulled, the trial marriage was kept secret, and the woman was free to try and marry another man. Of the offspring, only sons could continue the family's traditional cult, since when daughters married, they renounced their family and their father's cult. They now belonged to their husband's family and religion. Hence, family and cult were continued only through the sons.

The legislation of Augustus allowed widows and divorced women to remarry in order to have children. The aim of these laws was to obtain the greatest number of offspring in society. Augustus' birth rate laws indicated that a citizen had to have at least three children to be able to take possession of an inheritance. He had to impregnate his wife, even if it was achieved by different methods, so it was not rare for a Roman citizen to divorce his fertile wife to favour a childless friend. This is the case of Cato Uticensis who divorced his pregnant wife Marcia so that she could marry his friend Hortensius who still had no heirs (Knibiehler, 2001) Today this would be considered a prenatal adoption. The law also stated that if the husband died when his wife was pregnant, the unborn child was considered his father's heir.

The French anthropologist Héritier-Augé (1992) notes that donation of children was practised in many societies by distributing children among the wives of a polygamous husband so that infertile women, or those whose children had died, could access motherhood.

The Romans practised something similar to surrogate motherhood. A man whose wife was fertile could lend or rent her temporarily to someone who had no children. It was an agreement between men, as Héritier-Augé (1992) notes in which women had no say.

This brief historical overview of philosophical and scientific ideas about fertility reveals its central relevance in the androcentric and patriarchal social contract in ancient times. The female body was considered a means of reproduction from a utero-centric perspective, and women's subjectivity had no place in society. This leads us to think about the heritage, especially the patriarchal and androcentric heritages, which are part of present-day culture, in some areas as prejudice but in others playing a key role in society.

The Judeo-Christian heritage

In the Judeo-Christian heritage, marriage and conjugal love were oriented towards reproduction and the upbringing of children. Children were the ultimate gift of marriage and contributed to the parents' well-being, methods of birth control being penalised depending on the religion. Onanism as a contraceptive method was banned, considered illicit, and a sin. A Levirate Law forced the brother of a childless deceased husband to marry his widow. The first biblical case describing this law was that of Tamar and we also find the story of Rut (Nash, 1977). In this way, the widow did not remarry a man external to the family, and their first child would be named after the deceased brother, thereby perpetuating his name.

In Old Testament stories, children are a blessing. The aim of marriage, according to the ancient Hebrews, was to give birth to a son, who became the heir and continued the family line. Infertility was associated with a curse or divine punishment, and incest and adultery were not penalised when their aim was to repair infertility. The church did not inflict punishment on infertile women; they had to resign themselves to the divine plan and devote their time to doing good deeds or raising orphan children. Infertility did not justify spousal separation nor did it allow the husband to have a concubine.

In Biblical accounts, childless marriages such as those of Sarah, Hannah, and Rebekah are solved through divine intervention. In this sense, in Christian culture, motherhood is supra-natural and fertility is a God-given grace.

Historically, the rules of filiation depend not on a natural order but rather on shared beliefs within each culture. As stated by Héritier-Augé, social matters cannot be reduced to biology, nor can filiation be reduced to procreation (Héritier-Augé, 1992).

From the 11th century on, the so-called rural society was organised. Until the 18th century, the mother's role, practices, and representations were practically unchanged. Motherhood was considered a matter for women, who dealt with childbirth and the early education of their children. The mother was still considered inferior and subordinated to the man (Knibiehler, 2001), marriages were consummated to have children, and people commonly performed rituals to favour fertility. When pregnancy was delayed, the wife was considered solely responsible. It was then time for her to turn to miraculous springs, magical practices, pilgrimages, and devotions (Knibiehler, 2001).

In these societies, lineage was established through the women, and fatherhood was not part of the notion of naturalness. The father was the head of the family as a product of his rights.

During the Renaissance, a dissociative view of women was maintained: on the one hand, she was depicted as inferior and on the other, she was seen as a seductive courtesan. This era is the beginning of courtly love.

The human embryo

A story lies behind the image of the ovum and the spermatozoon giving rise to the human embryo, so well known to us at present. Feminist anthropologist Emily Martin (1994) notes that it is interesting to consider the possibility that culture may shape the way in which biologists describe their discoveries in the natural world.

In 1650, a major event took place: Harvey discovered that the human embryo develops from an egg, in the same way as mammals. This fact was proven by his disciples. Hence, the embryo developed from an egg, and women produce an ovum that was fertilised by men's sperm. A few years later, in 1677, van Leeuwenhoek and his assistant, Ham, discovered spermatozoa. However, Hartsoeker argued that sperm contained a homunculus: a minuscule, fully formed human being (Martin, 1994).

This established that women produce an egg that is fertilised by men's sperm. In this way, the role of women and men in reproduction was equated, overturning the prevalent theories of Hippocrates, Aristotle, Plato, and Galeno, who assumed exclusive participation by men. Based upon these findings, both men and women have the same responsibility in fertilisation (Giberti, 1992).

Martin (1994) notes that as she was learning more about the ovum and the spermatozoa, this knowledge was accompanied by descriptions linked to male and female stereotypes of each era. The ovum is seen as something large and passive that neither moves nor travels; it is instead transported or dragged through the fallopian tubes. Conversely, spermatozoa are smaller and are constantly active, travel at great speed, and have strong tails. This author quotes Gerald and Helen Schatten who compare the role of the ovum to that of Sleeping Beauty, seen as a sleeping bride waiting for her lover's magical kiss that will instil the spirit and bring her back to consciousness (Schatten and Schatten, 1984, cited in Martin, 1994).

In this view, the specific role of women is revalued, unlike her condition as being weak, cold, and moist in temperament compared to men's temperament, described as warm and dry.

Jean de Liébault (Tubert, 1991), Harvey's contemporary, argues that the uterus is the noblest and necessary part of women, its generating function constituting women as such. He revalues female qualities, but also reinforces the myth of the woman = uterus that dominates nineteenth-century gynaecology.

From a psychoanalytic perspective, we reflect on the way this uterocentrism exists in the concept of hysteria as the female illness par excellence. Although women are revalued in their reproductive role, their sexuality is repressed as part of the bourgeois order.

In the mid-twentieth century, Marie Langer (1951), in her book *Maternidad y sexo* [*Motherhood and Sex*] argues that in Freud's Vienna women suffered restrictions in the sexual and social spheres. However, they were encouraged to develop their maternal role and activities, and there was a prevalence of hysterical disorders. She poses that in the twentieth century, women acquired greater freedom in the social and sexual sphere, but psychosomatic disorders of the reproductive system increased, thereby giving rise to a conflict between motherhood and sex.

References

De Coulanges, F. (2020). *La ciudad antigua*. Colombia: Temis.

Giberti, E. (1992). "Mujer, enfermedad y violencia en medicina. Su relación con cuadros psicosomáticos." In Eds E. Giberti and A. M. Fernández, *La mujer y la violencia invisible* (p. 227).

Héritier-Augé, F. (1992). "Del engendramiento a la filiación." *Revista de psicoanálisis con niños y adolescentes*, (3), 22–31.

Knibiehler, Y & Fouquet, C. (1983). *La Femme et les Médecins* (Woman and Phisicians]. Paris: Hachette.

Knibiehler, Y. (2001). *Historia de las madres y de la maternidad en occidente*. Buenos Aires: Nueva Visión.

Lévi-Strauss, C. (1979). Antropología Estructural. Mito, Sociedad. *Humanidades*.

Langer, M. (1951). *Maternidad y sexo: estudio psicoanalítico y psicosomático* [*Motherhood and Sex. Psychoanalytic and Psychosomatic Study*]. Buenos Aires: Paidós.

Martin, E. (1991). The egg and the sperm: How science has constructed a romance based on stereotypical male-female roles. *Signs: Journal of Women in Culture and Society*, *XVI*(3), 485–501.

Martin, E. (1994). "La historia de un idilio científico." *Rev. Orgyn*, Bs.As., (3), 9.

Nash, D. (1977). *Goddesses, Whores, Wives, and Slaves: Women in Classical Antiquity*.

Schatten, G, & Schatten, H. (1994). "The energetic egg," *Medical World News*, 23K 51-53, In E. Martin, "La historia de un idilio científico," *Rev. Orgyn*, Bs.As., n°3, p. 9.

Tubert, S. (1991). *Mujeres sin sombra* [*Women without a Shadow*]. Madrid: Siglo XX.

Chapter 6

Fertility Myths and Rituals

Some notes on fertility rituals and myths

Motherhood and its counterpart, infertility, have been central issues in different cultures, expressed through various rituals and myths. For example, in agricultural societies numerous rituals promoted fertility: stones capable of fertilising the woman who touched them or waters with fertilising power. We may recall that in these societies, the fertility of the land, the livestock, and the arrival of children laid the foundations for survival of the social group. Infertility, its counterpart, was equated with draughts, barren land, crop failure, and death.

Studies of prehistoric times show the female character of primitive deities, although the existence of a primal matriarchy has not been proven. In ancient Mesopotamia, the great Mother Goddess had a generative power for lands, livestock, and human couples. Women were the first priestesses who worshipped these deities (Tubert, 1991).

When the patriarchy was established, this conception shifted, and male deities ousted female deities. Motherhood was now associated with nature, and fatherhood was defined not as a biological relation but as a social and legal right (Tubert, 1991).

Goldman Amirav (1996) described, based on biblical texts, the shift from matriarchy to patriarchy whereby the Mother Goddess was replaced by the one God who was responsible for conceptions and miracles. She mentioned that all biblical mothers came from the Mesopotamian region since the patriarchs went to that area to look for women. In the Mesopotamian culture, women and their reproductive capacity were worshipped. During their menstrual cycle, they were considered to have special powers and were consulted. Thus, Sarah, Rebecca, and Rachel left the most advanced civilisation of the time, which had worshipped the female principle since time immemorial, to join men who belonged to tribes of nomadic herdsmen. Goldman-Amirav noted that when meeting Jehovah, the biblical God with male features, these women became infertile, deprived of the value that had been granted to biblical women through motherhood. Sarah, Rebecca, and Rachel were the first

DOI: 10.4324/9781003296713-10

accounts of infertile women in the Bible. It was only by the Creator's gift, through his divine intervention, that these women could become mothers. Goldman-Amirav's hypothesis is supported by the proposal God's supremacy was affirmed in this way. Jehovah showed his power in areas in which the Mother Goddess formerly prevailed: a young woman could be made infertile and an elderly wife was able to give birth; such was his divine power.

In Mesopotamian culture, the most advanced civilisation of the ancient world was an agricultural society where women formed a unit with the earth. It was organised around large cities where writing was practised, and mathematics and astronomy developed. In the early days, most deities were female. Nature embodied both the fertile land where the seed was buried so that it bore fruit as well as the heavens and other fertilising forces including rain. They practised ritual ceremonies to favour rain by taking sculptures of female deities to the fields so as to increase the fertility of the land and gather abundant harvests. These rituals were performed by women, thereby confirming the female principle that ruled the fertility of the soil.

This parallel between the earth and the generative female function shows that just as a woman bore children, she also made the land thrive. By the same token, infertile women were not allowed to engage in cultivating the land since they prevented seeds from germinating. The same was true for women who were menstruating, since they were considered to be in a period of infertility.

In Greek mythology, the myth of Demeter and Persephone associated the fertility of land and nature with the cycle of life and death. The story of Demeter and her daughter Persephone attempted to shed light on central questions in life by representing the annual loss of soil fertility and the apparent death of nature in winter. Persephone's descent into the underworld of Hades depicted not only the cyclical character of nature but also of life itself in relation to death. As with the seed, she is buried in the earth only to ascend to life in the shape of a plant. Demeter represented both the uterus and the grave, similar to the figure of the Pachamama. Persephone depicted rebirth and regeneration, which was also associated with the moon, the spring, and the underworld. She was the goddess of beginnings or creation, annually re-creating the world through the abundance of each spring and harvest. She was the sustaining power of life (Bernardo, 1991).

Different figures have represented fertility throughout history. In Egypt, the lotus was called *the wife of the Nile* since when the river rises, the flower covers its surface. It was a flower consecrated to Isis, a virgin mother. Her son, Horus, was born from a lotus flower after Osiris' death. By bathing in the waters of the Nile and immersing his genitalia, Osiris had granted the river his fertilising power. Hence, the waters and the lotus flower symbolised fertility.

In India as in Egypt, the lotus flower that grows in sacred lakes represents fertility, and the water in which it multiplies has the virtue of fighting infertility. Shiva, the third deity of the great Hindu trinity and god of fertility, is the one most often implored by infertile women. In Indonesia, any woman who gave birth to a child with an unknown father was killed. However, she could avoid death by saying that her child had been conceived by a spirit, in which case she was congratulated (Tubert, 1991).

The figure of Quetzalcoatl in Mexico was represented by a feathered snake in Teotihuacan. In Meso-America, the snake was associated with the reproductive powers of the land and fertility, considering that the snake yearly sheds its skin and regenerates a new one.

For the Mapuche culture in South America, the human placenta had negative magical powers. When thrown onto a crop field, the soil was made barren, especially if this was done at the full moon.

The amalgamation of the earth and the female body also translates into the myth of the goddess Pachamama, the supreme deity of the Peruvian Andes, and in the indigenous rituals in north-eastern Argentina and all the Quechua people. The Pachamama ritual consists of burying a clay pot containing cooked food, coca, alcohol, wine, cigarettes, and peanut brandy or "chicha" somewhere near the house to please the Pachamama. This female deity produces and procreates. Pacha means universe, world, time, and place; and Mama represents the mother, as the word suggests. It is a ceremony to invoke the fertility of the land (Avenburg and Talellis, 2008).

In the African tribe of the Nuer, women unable to bear children were considered to be in the male category. Fatherhood and motherhood were not associated with male and female genders, since among the Nuer, there were cases of female fatherhood. Héritier-Augé (1996) argued that anthropological research in this tribe had shown that the difference between male and female was not sex, but fertility. In this social context, a woman who was not a mother lost the attributes of her gender, her female role being transformed into a male role. In some villages, marriage was not considered to be complete until a child was born, and in the case of infertility, the contract was annulled and the bride's dowry returned. In certain tribes in Nigeria, a woman who had already given birth to a child brought a much higher price than a young virgin (Tubert, 1991). We may recall the story of Princess Soraya, abandoned by Shah Reza Pahlevi due to her infertility.

In these stories of myths and rituals, we see how the conception and birth of a child occur in the intersection between the biological and the social sphere, the human and the divine, and male and female lineage (Belmont, 1989). In this perspective, women are reduced to their reproductive capacity, a utero-centristic view that equates "woman" with "mother".

The myth of maternal love

Until the 16th century, societies considered motherhood a natural event: children were born and then nursed and raised by their mothers or wet nurses. Before the industrial revolution, the family was first and foremost a productive unit; hence, women exercised their maternal responsibilities along with other productive activities. The feudal household was a family unit with the objective of preserving assets and passing on the lineage. Boys joined the adult world of work too early, and men were responsible for their training as soon as they reached a certain age.

It was not until the 17th and 18th centuries that secularisation diminished the influence of the Church, Catholic traditions were questioned, and a new model of society was created. At this stage, motherhood gained great importance: women were still subordinated to men but were revalued as mothers.

In the 17th century, issues such as induced labour, induced abortion, therapeutic abortion, and Cesarean sections were discussed. Also, women in labour and their babies were assisted, obstetrics treatises were written, and doctors gradually replaced midwives, who had been in charge of deliveries up to that time. Knibiehler (2001) notes how the glorification of motherhood prevailed during the 19th and 20th centuries given that medicine, especially gynaecology and obstetrics, entered an age of progress.

Towards the end of the nineteenth and the early twentieth century, Ehrenreich and English (1984) studied the representations of women in medical discourse in the United States. Studies showed that medical ideas about women's health were not limited to considering risks associated with reproduction, pregnancy, and birth; they also found that all female functions were considered intrinsically ill. For instance, the absence of menstrual periods was considered a pathological period in a woman's life.

As a consequence of society's mass industrialisation, work ceased to be home-centred, thereby giving rise to new environments such as schools and factories. The family reduced its size and isolated itself (Martínez, 1993). In this shift in perspective, emotional support became the very purpose of the family; in this context, the wife-mother took on the central role of preserving the emotional stability of the family unit. It was the mother who bore the moral responsibility for the care and upbringing of the children.

The rise and exaltation of maternal love was constituted as a natural and social value. Not only were motherly feelings and attitudes promoted, but the image of women as mothers was also fostered. Rousseau's manuals bore witness to his times when he wrote that maternal love is heroic in nature and is willing to sacrifice itself for the children (Knibiehler, 2001).

Women managed an increasingly smaller household, which established the maternal ideal that was henceforth constitutive and specific to female identity (Abadi and Alkolombre, 1999). Motherhood acquired the character of women's natural role. This maternal ideal equated women with mothers and with nature, shaping a new female narcissistic base. Therefore, social discourse as a collective construction defined female desire as being maternal.

Until that time, the family had basically been founded on lineage and fili-ation. Women, dominated by men, yielded to the husband and father as the family authority. However, it was the wife and mother who became the dom-inant figure at the core of the family in terms of organisation. In this way, motherhood became a source of respect and rights for women, given that it was they who fed the children while education was provided by fathers (Tubert, 1991).

The ideal that maternal love is sacrificial and heroic has its origins in this concept of the maternal-female. Throughout the 19th century and the first half of the 20th century, motherhood still played a central role in women's lives. Wars and population decline highlighted the demographic problem and the importance of birth rates.

Two major periods regarding family organisation that governed differ-ent modes of union between men and women can be distinguished thus far, according to Roudinesco (2005). The first was the traditional family, whose main purpose was to ensure the transmission of patrimony and worship, in which marriages were arranged by parents. The modern family followed towards the end of the 19th century and into the mid-20th century, initiating an affective logic. Marriage reflected love between spouses, who reciprocated feelings and wishes. In this model, the child played a central role and was in the care of both parents. In the second half of the 20th century, a new model emerged: the contemporary family, also known as the "postmodern" family, which entails the union of two individuals for a variable period of time.

Along with shifts in the family organisation came radical changes in reproductive medicine. Oral contraception was introduced in the sixties and reproductive techniques in the eighties. Both scientific developments mod-ified the role of motherhood, the essential arrival of children, and power relations between men and women.

Throughout this historical overview, we see how motherhood and father-hood are not only a product of individual desire, but also respond to social determinants that institute practices and orient desires in men and women. They also bring to light the extent to which parenthood, based on a repro-ductive biological view, is oriented according to the dominant beliefs and ideologies of each era and culture, thereby determining different meanings of fertility and its counterpart, infertility.

This cultural heritage reveals the various contexts and resolutions when the woman is faced with the inability to conceive: expulsion from marriages in ancient times, resigned acceptance in Judeo-Christian culture, and the secularisation that has yielded to the medical sciences and has displaced midwives.

We see how many of these beliefs concerning the maternal role and infer-tility as its counterpart remain valid to this day. From a psychoanalytical point of view, we may reflect on the effect of discourses and mandates inter-woven into the singularity of the desire for a child.

Infanticide, incest, and infertility in the Oedipus myth

Psychoanalysis has found ways to exemplify the traits of neurosis observed clinically through myths and legends, given that they express unconscious desires in a way similar to dreams.

Freud borrows the Oedipus tragedy from ancient mythology to develop the nodular complex of neurosis in children and adults called the Oedipus complex. It describes a triangular relationship between mother, father, and child.

Sophocles tells the story of Oedipus Rex, condemned for murdering his father and marrying his mother, a fate predicted before his birth by the oracle. In his attempt to escape his fate, Oedipus finally experiences it. All the people suffer as a consequence of Oedipus' crimes, the fruits of the earth no longer grow and women are unable to bear children. Because of the criminal, the wrath of the gods was turned on the people of Thebes.

Freud analyses the vicissitudes of the Oedipus complex, parricide and incest being key points from the child's point of view. Aberastury (1984) notes that Freud evaded or repressed what parents feel or do in relation to their children. She highlights that the figure of Oedipus' father, Laius, is essential to understand his son's fate. In this regard, she suggests that there is a story prior to the birth of Oedipus that includes infanticide, incest, and infertility.

Laius lived in Thebes, where he was sentenced to banishment for excesses related to dissipated behaviour and suspicions of homosexuality. He took refuge in Pelops, where the king entrusted him with the education of his son Chrysippus. However, not only did Laius educate him but he also perverted him by initiating him into homosexuality. At the sacred Nemean Games, Laius kidnapped Chrysippus and thereby prevented the sacred worship of the dead, since this ceremony could only be performed by the king's son. Chrysippus' father, the king of Pelops, was enraged and cursed Laius: he shall never have a child, and if he had one, death shall come after him.

After a time, Laius married Jocasta and returned to Thebes. In the wake of the curse of the king of Pelops, Laius decided to consult the oracle of Apollo, who predicted he would die by the hands of his son and the latter would marry his own mother. Therefore, he avoided procreating to escape this prediction; however, Jocasta deceived him when he was drunk, and a child was born. Laius again tried to flee his fate and ordered his infant son to be killed. He was duly hung by his feet from a bush on Mount Cithaeron. Oedipus, which means swollen feet, was found by a herdsman and delivered to the king and queen of Corinth, who were unable to have children. Thus, Oedipus was raised by Polybus and Merope, the king and queen of Corinth.

Years later, a drunkard tells Oedipus at a banquet that the king and queen were not his birth parents, but when he enquired about this statement, they deny it. Still not satisfied with his parents' answer, Oedipus consulted the oracle of Delphos, who predicted that he would murder his father and marry his mother. Frightened by this fate, he fled Corinth and headed towards Thebes. At a crossroads on that journey, he met Laius and as a result of an argument, Oedipus killed him, not knowing he was his biological father. Later on, he met the Sphinx, a monster half lion and half woman, who gave riddles to travellers and killed those who could not solve them. Thebes was devastated by a plague, this very Sphinx, that caused infertility and threatened its inhabitants. Everything died, crops and livestock, and women became infertile.

Oedipus solved the riddle of the Sphinx and freed the people of Thebes from the monster. The hero was rewarded and became the king of Thebes by marrying Jocasta. Four children were born of this marriage: Polynices and Eteocles, Ismene, and Antigone.

According to the oracle's prophecies, the plague would disappear when the murderer of Laius was discovered. The tragedy was unveiled by the oracle, and Oedipus discovered it was he who had killed his father and betrothed his mother. When the truth was revealed, Jocasta hanged herself and Oedipus gouged out his eyes, blinding himself. He then left Thebes accompanied by his daughter Antigone.

As the story unfolds, we see that Laius and his homosexuality play an essential role in the myth when he kidnaps Chrysippus, the son of king Pelops. In Greek culture, this was extremely serious since the son was the heir to the throne and the only person who could carry on the family religion. Laius received the worst punishment for his acts: infertility, in this case, being deprived of the possibility of having children. Here, infertility as the oracle's threat and favourite punishment of the tragedy's characters takes on paramount importance: the curse of not having children that weighs on Laius and the inability to have children of the Corinthian king and queen (Polybus and Merope, Oedipus' adopted parents).

The absence of children shifts from exclusion to punishment and drives the protagonists to an impulsive tragedy. As has been noted, this tragedy begins with a plague that leads to infertility in women, the soil, and the fields.

The plague as the inability to conceive reminds us of Freud (1914) when he points out every individual's double existence: we in ourselves are our own end and, at the same time, we are a link in a chain.

References

Abadi, G., & Alkolombre, P. (1999). "Lo femenino maternal, una figura posible de lo traumático." Paper presented at the *XX Symposium de la Asociación Escuela de Psicoterapia para Graduados.*

Aberastury, A., & Salas, E. J. (1978) In *La paternidad* (pp. 83–110). Buenos Aires: Kargieman.

Avenburg, K., & Talellis, V. (2008). Para la tierra, para nosotros y para los otros: Usos del cuerpo en el ritual de la Pachamama. IX Congreso Argentino de Antropología Social.

Belmont, N. (1989). Propositions pour une anthropologie de la naissance. *Topique*, *43*(1), 7–18.

Bernardo, A. (1991). *Deméter y Perséfone. El mito de la transformación cíclica*. Buenos Aires: Editorial Gredos, Colección Mitología Femenina.

Ehrenreich, B., & English, D. (1984). *Brujas, comadronas y enfermeras*. Barcelona: La-Sal.

Freud, S. (1914). On narcissism: An introduction. In Ed. J. Strachey, *The Standard Edition of the Complete Psychological Works of Sigmund Freud*, Volume XIV. London: Hogarth Press.

Goldman-Amirav, A. (1996). "Mira, Yahveh me ha hecho estéril," en *Figuras de la madre*, S. Tubert, comp., Feminismos, Madrid, pág. 41.

Héritier-Augé, F. (1996). *Masculin/féminin. La pensée de la différence* [Masculin-Feminine. Thought the difference]. Paris: Odile Jacob.

Knibiehler, I. (2001). *Historia de las madres y de la maternidad en occidente*. Buenos Aires: Nueva Visión.

Martínez, E. R. (1993). "Hacia una crítica de la maternidad como eje de construcción de la subjetividad femenina en psicoanálisis." In *Las mujeres en la imaginación colectiva*, A. M. Fernández, Paidós, Bs. As.

Roudinesco, E. (2005). *La familia en desorden*. Buenos Aires: Fondo de Cultura Económica.

Tubert, S. (1991). *Mujeres sin sombra [Women without a Shadow]*. Madrid: Siglo XX.

Index

male 67, 101n5, 101n8; sexual potency
67; supra-natural and 138; treatments
75, 81–82, 108–109, 114–129
fertility rituals and myths 141–147;
incest 146–147; infanticide 146–147;
infertility in the oedipus myth
146–147; myth of maternal love
143–145
Finzi, S. V. 22
Fiorini, G. 16, 17
Flis-Trèves, M. 121
Frankenstein (Shelley) 114
Frankenstein ou les délires de la raison
(Vacquin) 114
Freud, A. 7
Freud, S. 32–33, 41, 44, 79, 101n23,
147; aetiology of neurasthenia 36n4;
anal-erotic libido 11–12; "Analysis
Terminable and Interminable" 28;
Beyond the pleasure principle 98;
concept of drive 63; *Constructions
in analysis* 100; double existence 22;
Femininity 7; *His Majesty the Baby*
51, 53; hypotheses related to the
desire for a child in women 12; "The
Infantile Genital Organization"
9; initial masculine position 13;
on libido 9; on mourning 74; *On
Narcissism: An Introduction* 18,
63–64; on Oedipus complex of young
girl 10, 12, 13, 14, 28, 146; perspective
on female infertility 21; perspective
on female sexuality 8; phallic monism
13; on puberty 8; view on women's
psychosexual development 15
Freudian theory 45
Frydman, R. 24; *Les procréations
médicalement assistées: vingt ans
après* 107; *L'irrésistible désir de
naissance* 121, 122

Galeno 139
gamete donation 119–120
gamete intra-fallopian transfer (GIFT)
101n17
Garma, A.: *Psicoanálisis de los sueños
[Psychoanalysis of dreams]* 99
gender theories 2, 17, 20, 30, 46
genetic kinship 126
gestational surrogacy 125
Gilmore, D. D. 27
Glocer Fiorini, L. 46–47
Goldman-Amirav, A. 141–142

good enough mother 44
Greece 135–136
Green, A. 27, 28, 41–42, 52, 63; normal
maternal madness 43; *Passions et
destins des passions* 57n1
Groddeck, G. 31
Guerin, G. 21; *The Inconceivable Child*
114
gynaecological laparoscopy 101n17

Hassoun, J. 35
Héritier-Augé, F. 18, 22, 106, 107,
137–138, 143
Hippocrates 136, 139
Hippocratic Corpus 135
His Majesty the Baby (Freud) 51, 53
homosexuality 30, 146, 147
Horney, K. 13
human embryo 139–140
Huxley, A.: *Brave New World* 105
hysterectomy 79, 80, 101n14, 127, 130n8
hysteria 15, 25, 63, 140

identity 64, 109, 144; child 1; gender 27;
human 116; life goals and 21; love and
48; masculine 27, 34, 35; sexual 94
imaginarise 65, 71, 73, 122
imposed paternity 109–110
incest 146–147
The Inconceivable Child (Guerin) 114
individual treatment 117–118
infanticide 146–147
"The Infantile Genital Organization"
(Freud) 9
infertility 112; castration threat in 22;
enigmatic 83–90, 116; erogenous
body in 63–71; female 20–27; grief
54; male 32–36; in the Oedipus myth
146–147; permanent 79–80; transitory
80–82, 102n16
intracytoplasmic sperm injection (ICSI)
118–119, 129n2
intrauterine insemination 102n19
intrauterine insemination (IUI) 50, 80,
101n2, 102n19
in vitro fertilisation (IVF) 57, 101n20

Janaud, A. 51; *L'enfant a tout Prix [The
Child at Any Price]* 47, 119
John, E. 107
Jones, E.: on young girl unconscious
knowledge of vagina 13
Judeo-Christian heritage 138–139

telepathy 33
temporality 25–27
Testart, J. 106, 121
Török, M. 15
Tort, M. 22, 24, 106, 115
transference, body in 73–74
transitory infertility 80–82
transparent bodies 71–73
Tubert, S. 17, 48, 51; *Mujeres sin sombra: maternidad y tecnología [Women without a Shadow: Motherhood and Technology]* 15–16

ultrasound of the mind 112–113
uncanny dream 96–100
unresolved mourning 76–79
urgent decision 92–94

Vacquin, M. 120; *Frankenstein ou les délires de la raison* 114
varicocele 65, 67, 100n1, 101n6

Viennese Movement 15
virility 27, 28, 34, 35, 36, 48, 66, 119

Warnock, M. 130n7
Whitehead, M. 105
Winnicott, D. W. 44, 112; good enough mother 44
women: body 64–66; desire 7–20; expectations 119; health of 144; inferiority 136; menopause 79; motherhood in 95; psychosexual development 15
World War II 123

XY: On Masculine Identity (Badinter) 34

young girl: femininity 9; Oedipus complex in 10, 14; primary masculinity 13; unconscious knowledge of vagina 13, 17